28 Day Chair Yoga for Seniors to Lose Weight

Reclaim Your Strength, Flexibility, and Independence with Simple Exercises in Just Minutes a Day! + BONUSES

Carol Bolden

Table Of Content

Introduction

There once lived a lady by the name of Carol in a little town tucked away in the middle of the countryside. At seventy-two, she was a lively woman who liked to spend her days in her garden and going on long walks in the forests nearby. But as time passed, Carol developed several health problems that made her feel frail and unsteady. Her joints were rigid and inflexible, and her formerly powerful muscles had become weak. She could no longer enjoy the things she used to love to do, and it seemed like her body was betraying her.

Carol came to the realization one day as she was sitting in her garden and watching the sunset that she couldn't go on living this way. She didn't know where to start, but she needed to find a method to get her strength and flexibility back. That's when she thought of Mary, her close friend who had just begun doing chair yoga. Mary had encountered comparable problems, but she had managed to get over them.

Hopeful, Carol contacted Mary and requested her assistance. Mary was delighted to introduce Carol to the world of chair yoga and share her newly acquired expertise. Together, the two friends would sit in the yard and work through their aches and pains with slow, deliberate motions and breathing techniques.

Carol saw that her flexibility and strength were returning as she kept up her chair yoga sessions. She could feel her joints becoming more flexible and her muscles becoming stronger. She was walking through the woods again without feeling tired, the stiffness that had earlier troubled her slowly dissipating.

Carol realized that she had discovered the answer to her issues one day while relaxing in her garden. She was free to enjoy her life to the fullest again, having recovered her freedom. She realized she had to impart her newfound wisdom to others who were going through similar struggles while she enjoyed the warm light of the sun.

Carol set out to write a thorough manual on chair yoga with a strong sense of resolve in her heart. She devoted several hours to studying and trying out various methods so that she could write about her own experiences in the book.

Carol could not suppress a grin as she completed her book. She was aware that she had produced something unique in the form of a manual that would enable others to regain their fortitude, adaptability, and independence. She was sure the book would have a positive impact on readers' lives since she had put her whole being into it.

Carol released her book "28-Day Chair Yoga for Seniors to Lose Weight" with a feeling of joy and success. She gave it to her neighbors, relatives, and friends, and soon the news got out about her amazing guide.

Carol soon started to receive messages from individuals expressing gratitude for the great influence her book had had on their lives, coming from all over the globe. They told each other tales of how, like her, they had recovered their power and flexibility. They informed her that they felt more autonomous and in charge of their life and that they could now participate in their favorite hobbies.

Upon hearing these tales, Carol was ecstatic and realized that her work had had an impact. She kept up her daily chair yoga practice and expressed her gratitude for the gift of a second shot at life that it had given her.

Therefore, my dear reader, don't give up if you encounter similar difficulties. Chair yoga is a simple but effective exercise that offers hope. Carol's narrative demonstrates that you can always regain your strength, adaptability, and self-sufficiency. Turn the page to start your trip, that's it.

Remember, the book "28 Day Chair Yoga for Seniors to Lose Weight" has the answer to your issue right here. So, settle in, take a seat, and let's get started.

The Benefits of Chair Yoga for Seniors

Exercise is known to have many advantages that continue far into old age, but doing high-intensity exercises as your body gradually deteriorates is risky. There is a greater chance of discomfort and harm, and healing takes longer. You may strengthen your body generally without running the danger of strains by practicing yoga. Since chair yoga makes use of a chair for support, let's explore the various advantages of yoga for senior individuals. To put things in perspective, chair yoga is ideal for those who have vertigo, arthritis, movement problems, and more.

Greater Adaptability

One of the many benefits of yoga is flexibility, and chair yoga is no different. Chair yoga pushes the body to push itself and helps to stretch areas of the body that may not ordinarily be stretched. This improves a person's general mobility for everyday chores by helping them become more flexible and maintain it.

Enhances Strength of Muscle

Chair yoga offers several positions that help strengthen and build muscles. This and flexibility work together to enhance mobility and balance. Gaining muscle can also aid in preventing injuries to your body.

Aids with coordination and balance

Chair yoga facilitates the transition of positions to increase your body's spatial awareness. You might feel more connected to your body by doing yoga, which trains your mind to concentrate on various body parts and use them to their fullest potential. You gradually get better coordination and balance training from this.

lessens tension

Yoga also improves your ability to concentrate on your breathing and physical alignment. This aids in detaching you from life's harsh situations. Yoga incorporates meditation as a means of relaxation and stress relief.

lessens discomfort and improves the ability to manage pain

When you exercise, a hormone called endorphins is produced, which not only improves your mood but also helps to reduce some of the pain and suffering. Chair yoga, sometimes referred to as the body's natural medicine, teaches you how to manage discomfort by focusing on your breathing.

Encourages More Restful Sleep

Regular exercise improves the quality of your sleep and aids your body's sleep-wake cycle. The same is true for chair yoga, which requires just the correct amount of energy expenditure without tiring the practitioner.

Enhances Self-Belief and Reduces Depression and Anxiety

Studies indicate that yoga, particularly chair yoga, may be able to reduce symptoms of anxiety and sadness in people of all ages. You may release bad emotions from life with the attention required for yoga, and you'll walk out of the practice feeling renewed and light.

Essential Equipment and Preparation

Essentials of at-home yoga to get started

You will need certain yoga equipment to practice yoga at home. Yoga's simplicity lies in the fact that you may practice it at home or on the go without a lot of equipment. The very least that you need is a mat. For a good at-home yoga practice, the additional things on our list of essentials are strongly advised. The necessities are arranged below in terms of usability and need, so start your shopping at the top and work your way down.

- Yoga mat: A yoga mat costs around $15–25 and can be purchased online or at any big-box retailer. Quality matting keeps you from sliding and provides some cushioning against a hard surface. A standard mat should work just fine whether your flooring is carpeted or has another sort of flooring. If your home has hardwood flooring, you may want to acquire a thicker mat.

- Wear comfortable yoga attire: To begin, just put on what you would regularly wear to the gym or for running. Make sure your clothing allows you to freely move through the various yoga positions. Should you engage in more strenuous yoga practices, you should look for clothing that rapidly dries and wicks away perspiration. Above all, choose clothing that you are most at ease wearing.

- yoga blocksFor those just starting, yoga bricks or blocks made of wood, foam, or cork may be quite beneficial. When you are in poses that call for you to be grounded and balanced, you utilize them as an extension of your hands to steady your body. They cost around $13 for a pair of two and are available online or at most big-box shops. They are available in a variety of shapes and sizes.

- If you have limited flexibility in your legs, a yoga strap, also known as a yoga belt, maybe a very helpful tool. It serves as an extension of your arms, enabling you to maintain your balance and extend the position farther. Yoga straps cost around $7 and can be purchased online or at most big-box retailers.

- Yoga mat cleaning: A soiled yoga mat may become slick and stinky. To clean your mat, you can either manufacture your spray or purchase a pre-made one that typically costs approximately $11. All that is required to maintain the fresh appearance of your mat is a periodic fast spritz and wipe clean.

- Towel: If you do hot yoga or find that you perspire a lot while doing yoga, you need a microfiber yoga mat towel. Smaller microfiber hand towels may be used if just your hands are becoming sweaty and slick. To keep yourself dry and clean, make sure the towel is sufficiently thick and absorbent.

Essentials for seasoned yogis practicing at home

- Yoga blanket or bolster: You will need one or two yoga blankets and a bolster for restorative positions. Although you may use any spare blankets, folded towels, and firm cushions you have lying around your house, it will be ideal to have the right props to support you in these passive poses if you routinely practice restorative yoga.

- Meditation cushion: When practicing sitting meditation, you need to provide support under your hips to support your whole body. This may be accomplished with a bolster or yoga blanket, but if you often meditate, it is preferable to utilize a cozy meditation cushion to sit on during your sitting poses. Cushions are available in a variety of sizes and forms; to choose the ideal one for you, see our information on meditation cushions.

- Foam roller: Before or during your yoga practice, you may wish to use a foam roller to gently massage and release tension from stiff and tight muscles. Choose a foam roller depending on your body type, preferred style of massage, and price range. Foam rollers come in a wide variety of forms and sizes.

- Yoga balls or wheels are wonderful props to experiment with if you like backbends and restorative yoga. It may also be used to increase the difficulty of certain positions. As an alternative, an inflatable yoga ball is a fantastic tool for core strengthening activities and for supporting backbends.

- When you're resting in a Shavasana stance, you may use a weighted eye cushion to ease the tension around your eyes and encourage deeper levels of relaxation.

Components of a peaceful yoga area

- Locate a spotless, cozy area in your house where you may practice in silence. A few simple things placed in your area may make a big difference in how much you appreciate and have fun.

- Air Fan: To stay cool and comfortable throughout your practice, you may wish to invest in a tiny, portable fan if you tend to become hot and sweaty.

- Portable heater: Instead of heating the whole home, you may use a portable heater to warm up your yoga room if you love hot yoga classes or live in a chilly region.

- Aroma diffuser: Lighting incense or using an essential oil diffuser can further enhance the environment in your practice. Depending on the atmosphere you want to create, you may use different smells to make your environment more energetic or peaceful.

- Bluetooth speaker: You may enhance the audio quality of any music or audio instructions you use in your practice by using a high-quality speaker.

Shopping advice for yoga necessities

- To get the greatest offers and pricing, shop around. If you're new, you may want to check out discounted yoga sets that come with a mat, blocks, straps, and other accessories.

- Seek for natural and eco-friendly materials such as organic cotton, cork, and rubber.

- Find out from your other yogis what companies and products have enhanced and supported their yoga practice the most.

- Investing in cheaper gear initially and then upgrading to better quality stuff after you've had more time to get a feel for things can be the best course of action if you're not sure how serious and devoted you will be.

DAY 0

Greetings and thank you for buying my book, 28 Day Chair Yoga for Seniors to Lose Weight. I'm Carol, and I'm so glad you could join me today. We're going to embark on a 28-day chair yoga journey together. Sometimes, when beginning any kind of commitment, it's a good idea to connect and give it your all. Over the next 28 days, we'll experience our chair yoga practice as a community, which is incredibly powerful. First, if you've never done chair yoga before, this 28-day series will set you up for success.

If you've been with me for some time, you may be thinking that I want to go back to the basics, but I encourage you to embrace the process and reap the rewards of letting go of your preconceptions. All you need is comfortable clothing that doesn't restrict your movement; you can choose to wear tennis shoes or go barefoot. When I teach in person, we usually wear shoes.

I advise against wearing sandals. You know, you can't just slip your feet about in them. To prevent the chair from sliding, you'll also need a stable chair with no arms or wheels. You can also place the chair on a carpet or a sticky mat, such as a yoga mat, to keep it stable. This way, if you're pushing on the chair while standing, you can be sure it won't slide out from under you. In our chair yoga practice, we perform all the same poses, or asanas, that you would perform in a matte yoga practice.

The difference is that instead of getting up and down from the floor, we will either be seated in our chairs or stand the entire time. If you prefer, you can remain seated. We occasionally use yoga blocks or straps; if you don't have any, you can make do with a large book, a necktie, or a scarf. These can be helpful because the block is used to pull the floor or perhaps the chair seat closer to us, and the strap extends our arm's length.

However, I'm here to tell you that if you don't have any of these, you can still complete the work without them. The last thing you'll need is those selections, which I swear I'll always provide you. I understand that you value your time and am grateful that you have chosen to spend some time with me. You have my commitment that you will dedicate some time each day to practicing these chair yoga poses, which are very powerful. Share this with your loved ones so they can respect the time you've set aside for yourself and be empowering. Better yet, invite them to join you.

Thus, salutations to my fellow seniors I'm so glad you could join me for this beautiful chair yoga journey. Please take a seat back in the chair, place your hands on your thighs with the palms facing up, and inhale deeply. As you exhale, consider what you hope to gain from this journey together. You can also close your eyes or soften them. Inhale deeply and exhale once more, bringing your hands to your heart and your mind. As you do so, honor one another by saying namaste. Then, return your hands to your thighs and open your eyes.

I appreciate you joining my group, whether you found me later in life or started this trip in the new year, on this investigation of chair yoga.

Just know that it's a lovely method to show yourself respect. Tomorrow, I'll see you.

DAY 1

On the first day of our 28-day chair yoga adventure, we will remain seated and concentrate on our breathing. We will now begin by sitting up straight and pushing forward in our chair so that we are not reclining at this point. As we begin each practice, we'll take some time to focus on these three elements as a way to help center our minds and get ready for our practice.

Next, we're going to focus on our position in the chair. First, I want you to place both of your feet on the floor. We're thinking about grounding our feet. If you've chosen to wear tennis shoes, you can still feel your feet inside the shoes as they ground to the Earth. Remember that those shoes do provide a lot of stability and support, so feel free to wear them.

I just wouldn't recommend sandals okay so your feet don't just slide around in them too much so again we're going back to our grounding our feet to the Earth so so the grounding in yoga is connecting to the Earth both physically and emotionally so as we feel both of our feet as they connect to the Earth we make sure that they're flat on the floor and equally weighted so many of us pronate or supinate our feet when we walk it's just kind of sometimes it's sort of natural but I just want you to think right now make sure that each of those pressure points and what I'm referring to like when I talk about those pressure points is there's one point behind the big toe there's one point behind the little toe and there's two points of the heel and I want you to feel all four of those pressure points on each foot on the floor and equally weighted okay so kind of got that down.

Now the next thing we're going to think about is connecting to our chair so we refer to this as grounding our sits bones now the sits bones also called sitting bones they refer to the bottom part of the pelvis and we're going to do just a little exercise to better feel that area of the pelvis okay so the first thing I want you to think about sitting on your hands Palms up, all right?

Now, we're going to raise one hip, place our palms palm up on the chair, and place our pelvis there. As you sit there, you'll notice that the pointy bones are there.

We're going to perform a little exercise to help us feel those moving bones. hence the hip hints Here are those sharp hip bones. I would want you to rock them in the direction of your shoulders.

Notice how the sits and bones sort of moved back. Now, we're going to move those hip tips in the direction of our shoulders. Notice how they go forward. Let's do it again. hip-tips I said, "Okay, let's do this again," gesturing to our shoulders and my mentor's legs. You may now feel your sit bones shifting backward toward your shoulders. Let's repeat it a few more times. I'm not cueing that well, am I? Hip tips towards your knees. What am I doing wrong here? Hip tips to shoulders. You'll feel them sliding forward. Hip tips to back. I apologize, but I believe you are sensing it.

I think I've got my shoulders and my knees mixed up there that's okay you got the sensation don't you yeah all right so now what I want you to do is come back with that crown of that head nice and tall and I want you to remove the hands now do you feel those those pointy bones do you feel those sits bones and how you're sitting up nice and Tall on top of them so kind of wherever you're Landing when you're sitting nice and Tall that should be right on those sits bones and I want you to feel those connecting to the chair and feeling that they're equally weighted now we're going to lift our heart nice and tall and let's lower those shoulders down out of the ears this is another thing you'll hear me talk about quite a bit shoulders out of the ears so as we lift our heart almost inevitably those shoulders want to come with and I want you to really think about pulling those shoulders down we're going to place our hands lightly on our thighs flip those Palms up towards the ceiling now close your eyes and if you don't want to close your eyes that's fine just soften your gaze look down just don't let the head be the thing to fall right I want you just to have that the Gaze down I'm going to close my eyes.

Now I want you to focus on your heart center so we're just connecting inward and we're feeling that breath so we've got our body connected to the chair we're breathing our natural inhalation and exhalation and we're focusing our mind or our consciousness on that Heart Center just feel that natural breath feel the rhythm of the breath let's do that one more time just a natural breath We're going to raise our hands to our hearts and declare our goals for the practice today. Just concentrate on the goal you have in mind, then bring your hands back down to your thighs and open your eyes to assess how you're feeling. We're going to begin every practice in a very similar way, so maybe you're feeling calm or relaxed.

Either way, it's a pretty good feeling, isn't it? Okay, so now we're going to move into a little series here to stretch our neck. We're going to drop our right ear towards the right and hold this for just a few breaths, feeling like we're giving that neck a little bit of time to stretch right just a little bit. Next, we're going to drop our chin towards our chest and then we're going to drop that left ear towards that left shoulder.

Ah, does that feel good Let's bring our chins up to our chests—I like it. Subsequently, we will examine the rim from the front, center, and rear. We'll roll our shoulders as well.

This is one of those exercises where I want you to think about executing it with awareness. Let's take those shoulders down, back, up, and forward. Why is it happening? What feelings are there? Let's go in that way one more time. While I'm doing this, I'm focusing on how everything feels and what's going on in my body. In the end, we'll flip it over, which will be a great way to loosen up the shoulders and even the neck a little.

Gorgeous One More Time and release it and I don't know if you noticed but I went pretty slowly so that's the other thing I think if you do those pretty fast you might not get the same Sensations as doing it slowly so my preference is to do those pretty slow so that's you know what what I prefer to do so the next pose is called Mountain pose and again this is another pose we'll do in most practices it's just a nice way to begin to lengthen through the spine as we warm things up so we're going to bring our hands down by our side and I like to spread my fingers wide so it just gives those hands a little stretch you see what I'm doing there I'm just spreading those fingers now if that doesn't feel good for you or if you've got arthritis in your hands or whatever and you don't want to do it then don't do it it's okay I'm just going to do that because I like to stretch my fingers a little bit okay so now we're going to move those arms up now you'll hear me refer to this position right here in a couple of different ways it's I call it gold post arm so think about football right if you're a football fan you might kind of see the goal post here it's also referred to as goddess arms so you might hear me call it goddess arms It's the same pose, but I want you to focus on lifting up through your chest and pulling your shoulders down out of your ears.

Squeeze your shoulder blades back behind you to make it an active pose. Instead of just hanging here with our arms in the air, we're actively pulling the shoulders down out of your ears. Next, we'll lengthen our fingers by extending two fingertips toward the ceiling, and then we'll enter an extended Mountain pose. Okay, so your shoulders are down and your arms are extended, but I want you to consider trying to touch the ceiling with your fingertips while simultaneously pulling the shoulders down.

This will engage your abdominals, so pull that belly in. We're going to repeat our mountain pose, so let's come down and spread our fingers wide. You can feel it proceed after arms Goddess arms bring your shoulders down, pushing them back behind you, tightening your fingers to the ceiling, and extending into your spine. Alright, how did that feel? Do you want to roll your shoulders again? I'm all about rolling those shoulders so anytime you want to do that that's fine. Inhale deeply, then exhale completely.

What was your impression of the mountain pose? The next pose is the Staff Pose. This is one of those poses where you'll think there's nothing to it until you do it. Then, you'll feel what's happening in your body, and it's pretty amazing how much you can feel without even looking like you're doing anything. To start, we'll place our hands right under our arms, right at the armpits. I want you to use your hands to cue your body to lengthen, lifting and lengthening through the spine, so we're using those hands to kind of pull ourselves up.

Next, we'll release our hands and just place them on the chair's seat, kind of back behind our hips. Do you feel that? There's more to that pose than meets the eye, so we're going to do some body circles this time. Um, this is a little bit of movement for the spine so we're going to take our hands on our thighs and that's going to give us some really good support okay so we're going to start in One Direction, and make some big old circles so I'm going to go to the right a little. You have to use your abdominals here to keep this position. I know right, one more breath and release, can we do that once more just for fun? Alright, okay, ready, let's do it. In the same way maybe take a breath in As you go forward and exhale As you move back, if you'd like, we can start adding in a little bit of breath. I'll tell you that as we go, let's stop and reverse before I start talking.

Let's reverse so that I can tell you that if you add in the yoga breath at any point and you feel unwell, dizzy, or like it just doesn't work for you, just breathe normally. I'll cue you to add the yoga breath, but you don't have to feel compelled to do so. Let's do one more: we're inhaling forward and exhaling back. Okay, let's all get seated. How did that feel? We're beginning to move into that spine a little bit right now, but having the hands on the thighs Alright, so the next exercise is a little knee rotation. To do this, I'll grab my right knee, bring it up, and gently squeeze it. This is going to be extremely gentle.

Next, I'm going to reach behind my thigh and rotate back and forth, up, and down, just to give my hip joint a little more openness and movement. Maintaining the hip joint's range of motion at all times is a great concept, so let's turn it around. You seem to be OK. Okay, are we prepared to begin those rotations so that we may go sufficiently out and across? You already know that we will travel both ways, so it's okay if you choose to begin in the other direction. Let's now turn our circle around. only moving that little hip joint a little bit on today, the first day of our 28-day adventure.

We're going to go to the other side, so let's place that leg down. If it seems comfortable, hold your shin and pull. You're going to merely grip behind the thigh and pull if it hurts your knee. It's OK, so never do anything that causes pain. We are going to return to the goddess stance of sitting. Do you recall how we began earlier, in the embrace of the goddess? We're going to give those legs a bit more breadth now. We will extend upward through the head's crown and toward the ceiling. Squeeze your shoulder blades back together as you raise your arms and bring them back behind you.

Pose is God. We are left with one breath. We are going to put our hands up to our thighs now, listen. Then, I'd want you to simply let your feet drop to the side. This one seems okay. Now, are we prepared to carry out the whole process again? This is the moment to bring our hands back down to our thighs and give those knees one more fold. Let's go back into those goddess arms and spread those knees. Remember to squeeze your shoulder blades back behind you and raise your head. Extend your arms in a goddess manner, squeeze your shoulder blades back, inhale at this point, then bring your hands to your thighs, bend your knees, and experience the rotation once again. We will heel-toe those feet back together to get into the shavasana stance after opening the knees.

Let's take a seat back in our chair and recline back; this is our last relaxation posture. Gently put your hands on your thighs if that is comfortable. After that, raise your hands toward the ceiling. Inhale deeply, then exhale. As you release the air, soften or shut your eyelids. Proceed to finish the position. Although it will need time and work, the rewards will be great. No matter how many justifications you come up with, none of them will solve the problem or achieve the goal. Your exertion is what will make the difference.

You will prevail even though it will take a while to fight—you'll be pushing uphill and against a strong wind. You'll gain confidence and strength. In the near term, you'll have some excellent momentum and something to show for the time that has passed, so it's simpler to put things off, postpone, give in to doubt, and hesitate. Nevertheless, if you take a comprehensive approach, it will become clear that your best bet is to go on with completing it now, while your drive is strong. But when you've made the first step, you should keep moving forward until you can reflect on it and be happy that you did.

Take a deep breath, then release it all. Pull on the head gently, elevate your right hand, drop your right ear to your right shoulder, open your eyes, and press your left hand to the floor before releasing it. Raise your hands, chin to chest, and pull lightly on your head so that your elbows fall to the floor and release it. The left ear should move in the direction of the left shoulder.

As the first day concludes, we greet one another with namaste. Congratulations, my bottoms-down friends. Please keep coming; I think the toughest thing is simply getting to the chair. Gently pull on the head with your left hand while you bring your right hand down to the floor to release it. If you wish to extend your jaw, look outside and gently expand your mouth.

DAY 2

Today, as we begin our 28-day Chair Yoga journey.

So let's get started so we're going to start by sitting up nice and Tall we're going to move forward in our chair we're not leaning back so if you remember from day one that we'll start our practice by focusing on the mind and the body and the breath so as we begin each practice we'll take a little bit of time to focus on these three elements we're going to take place both of our feet on the floor and we're going to ground them each foot to the Earth so if you remember from yesterday just make sure each foot is on the floor and that all four pressure points are equally weighted now if you tend to pronate or supinate it's very common just be mindful and try to get those feet flat on the floor now the next thing we'll do is ground our sits bone

so if you want to take a moment and sit on your hands again like we did yesterday and feel those moving up you know forward and back feel free to do so but I want you to land with those sits bones equally weighted on the chair and feel that grounded to the seat of the chair we're going to lift our heart lower our shoulders down out of the ears place the hands lightly on our thighs flip those Palms up close your eyes connect to your heart center and just feel your breath just your natural inhalation and exhalation feeling the rhythm of that breath connecting to the rhythm of the heart and the rhythm of the Mind bring your hands to your heart set your intentions for today's practice one more breath here bring your hands back down to your thighs and open your eyes ah we're gonna draw our shoulders up into those ears right I'm always saying pull the shoulders down out of the ears well right now we're going to draw them up and then we're just going to let them fall so we're kind of letting gravity help us there let's shrug those shoulders and

we're going to let them fall one more time shoulders up into the ears and we're just gonna let them fall ah excellent work so we're going to take our right arm and we're going to extend it out we're going to let our head fall the other so just a little different way to stretch into that neck so we're kind of pushing through the palm of this hand towards that wall beside us as we just let this head fall kind of ear to shoulders that makes sense yeah okay let's bring that hand down and bring the head up wow there's something about adding that extended R right okay we're going to do the other side so we're going to extend the arm and then let that head fall so just think about pushing through the palm of that hand to give that neck a little extra stretch oh yeah just one more breath here and then we're going to bring that hand down and then we're going to bring that neck up let's do one more shoulder shrug just for the fun of it shrug it and release ah all right excellent so we move back into our Mountain pose like we did yesterday okay so we're going to come into Mountain pose spread our finger fingers wide to stretch unless it doesn't feel good then don't do it right we're going to come to the scopo storms we're going to squeeze that shoulder blades back behind us now we're going to take our fingertips to the ceiling pull the shoulders down make sure your abdominals stay engaged here and we're stretching those fingertips up towards the ceiling extended Mountain pose bring their hands down we're going to do that again here we go spread those fingers I know goal post arms are you squeezing your shoulder blades back behind do you have your belly button in towards your spine that engage those abdominals up we go lengthening to the ceiling feel that stretch it's a very active pose right we're not just hanging out here we're stretching one more breath and

bring your hands down to your side okay so we're going to move into a pose it's it's their cat and cow and we often do these two poses together so we're going to bring our hands to heart all right and I want you to think about lifting through the spine crown of the head to the ceiling and opening up through the throat so I'm not really looking up that's not the idea but I do want the throat to be open so this is our starting position now we're going to move into cow pose first and this version we're going to bring our hands back behind us and grab the back of the chair now as you do that I want you to pull your shoulders down lift up through the heart and open through the throat you're going to look up just slightly okay do you feel that there's a little arch in the back belly stays tight now that those abdominals are what's going to protect that back okay so a little arch in the back all right are we

ready to move into cat's pose I know I'm not tired of being here too are we ready here we go so now as we move into cat pose I want you to think about pulling your ribs back that tailbone is going to go heavy you're going to round the spine and place your hands on the thighs so let the head fall what I'll see in my classes my in-person classes is people here you know they're holding their head up I want you to really think about tucking the chin and letting that head fall that's where you're going to maximize the stretch in the upper back and the neck okay so we're going to come back into cow pose again are we ready we're going to grab the back of that chair we're going to lift up open up through that throat let's add the breath inhale here exhale round down pull the ribs back tailbone heavy tuck the chin let the head fall there's your exhale let's do that a few more times we're going to lift up into cow pose opening up squeezing those shoulder blades behind inhaling here exhaling into cat's pose rounding the spine pulling those ribs back and one more final time adding that breath remember if you don't add the breath don't right just breathe naturally don't hold your breath just don't you don't have to

do that yoga breath and then round it down last one all right let's come back up into seated now we'll do that one a lot too because it's just a really good thing to warm up that spine so a little you know movement in that spine okay so we're going to move back if you were with me yesterday you'll remember we did that goddess pose so we're going to do goddess pose but we're going to do a little add-on and I hadn't mentioned this yet but in my classes I'll often do a pose and then we might add something on and you don't ever have to add on if you don't want to right you can just keep doing the previous version of the pose and it's fine so this is going to be our seated goddess and then we're going to add horse pose to it so we're going to start with our feet first so we'll do our heel toe heel toe so now my legs are a little bit wide okay let's go ahead and add our goddess arms we've learned how to do those we're going to squeeze those shoulder blades behind us goal post arms goddess arms okay now I'm going to lift my right heel up off the

floor so there's a little work for that calf and then we're going to put that heel down and then we're going to lift the other heel up there's that calf and we're going to put that down let's do the other side again lift and down lift and down let's go ahead and bring our hands down and if you remember from yesterday let's do that little internal hip rotation I just like that you know we don't internally rotate the hips very much it's not something that we just naturally think about doing and it's just an it's a good stretch okay so now we're going to bring those knees back open again we're going to come back to that those goddess arms okay so lifting up nice and Tall remember crown of the head to the ceiling squeeze your shoulder blades

back behind okay let's start with our left heel we're going to lift and lower right heel lifts and lower right heel lift and lower left heel lift and lower one more time lift and lower lived and lower again lift and lower lift and lower and let's bring our hands down and through the internal hip rotation so here's one more little thing about me I will say one more generally that means we've got to do one on each side so it's technically two more so just know that that whenever I say one more usually it's both sides okay and if I remember I say it but a lot of times I don't remember okay knees come up now we're going to do one more thing here before we add add one more thing on so this is our final add-on in this position all right are we ready getting ready for horse we're gonna lift one heel then the other heel both heels at the same time and then down and down now let's start with this one first lift and lift hold breathe and down and down okay are we ready let's lift lift

and lift hold breathe down and down one more lift and lift hold and breathe down and in our final add-on okay are we ready we're gonna lean our goddess do you feel your shot Oh, Matt I'm not sure whether you've heard, but I just had a backache. Who needs a chiropractor when you have yoga? We're going to climb, then lean the other way, and then twist—I'm not serious. First let's glance to the right, then to the center, and finally let's turn around. We will return to the center. We will lower our hands once again. Together, let their knees collapse. There's only one little tiny hip rotation left. What is the feeling on that? Okay, let's slide back into our chair's back. We are going to recline. We are going to enter shavasana, the

position of rest. You may recline and inhale and exhale deeply. Close your eyes or look away. boldness as well as affection Lead by example, show love, and bravely navigate each new situation. Consider how you may approach this from a place of love and bravery before you speak or act. You will likely need to take on more difficulties and work harder if you adopt this attitude, but you will be more aware of the things that really add richness and purpose to life. You'll be able to change the world for the better in a place where it seems like everything is always

going wrong. When fear and complacency overwhelm you, make the decision to live above the usual; allow life's sweetness to shine through in everything you say, do, and feel, and then bravely live that love out. Take a deep breath, release it all, and open your eyes. The right ear should move in the direction of the right shoulder. Lift your right hand. Gently pull the head while releasing and pushing your left hand down toward the floor. Lower your chin to your chest and gently pull the head with your hands reaching up. We greet each other with

namaste and have progressed to day two. As I've already indicated, getting to the chair is the toughest part, so please keep coming. Approach your left shoulder with your left ear down. With your left hand, extend upward. Apply the lightest subtug possible to the heads and then release them. If you want to extend your jaw, open your mouth.

DAY 3

today is day three of our 28 day chair Journey day three of our 28-day chair yoga journey together that's kind of hard to say and we're going to stay seated again today and we'll add on to our cat and cow poses and we'll add a little gentle twist

let's get started we're going to start by again sitting up nice and Tall moving forward in the seat we're not leaning back right so remember that we start our practice focusing on that mind and body and breath all right so lets Place both of our feet on the floor and we're going to ground each foot so think about those sits Bones on the chair the feet are on the floor equally weighted the sits bones are on the chair equally weighted now we're going to live that heart and we're going to lower our shoulders out of our ears Place their hands lightly on your thighs

flip the Palms up towards the ceiling close your eyes and connect feeling your natural inhalation and exhalation here connecting to that Heart Center we're letting go of everything outside of the room, focusing inward begin to elongate that breath little bit so we're going to inhale a little more deeply and exhale a little more completely so just a few like that checking in seeing how that's feeling and then just breathe normally feeling the rhythm of your natural breath as it connects to the rhythm of

your heart and the rhythm of your mind let's do the elongation again inhaling a little more deeply exhaling completely just a couple more like that one more just breathe your natural breath bring your hands to your heart and set your intentions for today's practice focusing in on what you want to accomplish one more breath here we're going to bring our hands back down to our thighs and open our eyes and let's roll our shoulders a little bit so just feeling that shoulder roll here

feeling all the sensations taking your time no worries and then let's reverse it just feeling that all those Sensations right so we're connecting that that brain with what our body is doing feeling all those Sensations okay very very good so we're going to go ahead and grab the back of our chair and I want you to lift through the heart and pull your shoulders back and then we're going to let our right ear fall to our right shoulder so this is a little different feeling stretch for that neck then we're going to drop our chin towards our chest and then we're going to do the other side and we're going to do chin to chest now let's release the back of the chair bring the hands back to the thighs and roll our shoulders again ah that should feel good I don't know for me I kind of like to move my head around just a little bit as well all right very very good okay moving on we're going to move into a mountain pose so we're going to come down bring our hands down by our sides spread those

fingers so we're going to be adding a little bit on here remember you don't ever have to add on if you don't want to add on it's fine let's come to those goddess arms those goalpost arms squeeze your shoulder blades back behind you now we're going to lengthen our fingers to the ceiling right now arms are nice and long pull those shoulders back down all right now here's our little add-on so we're going to bring our right arm down by our chair you can hold the chair if you wish you're going to lengthen

your left arm up towards the ceiling and then we're going to lean our Mountain one more breath here all right let's come up and we're gonna do that whole series again here we go Mountain pose go post arm squeeze fingertips to the ceiling now we're going to take our left hand to the chair right hand extends nice long and lean and up we go all right very very good okay so we're going to move back into our cat pose and our cow pose so remember let's bring our hands to Heart we're going to lift through the spine

and open up through the throat now as you move into your cow pose we're going to bring our hands back to the chair and we're going to lift through the throat right and then we're going to round down into our cat pose think about pulling the ribs back tailbone goes heavy round the spine let the head fall we're going to add the breath we're going to inhale come up into cow pose grab the back of the chair lifting exhale we're going to round down into cat's pose inhale we're going to lift into cow

pose and exhale into cat pose and let's release that okay very good so we're going to add on to our cat and cow pose it's just a wide arm okay so what we're going to do is bring our hands back behind our head and elbows are wide so it's the same idea so we're going to lift through the throat looking up slightly inhale here and then as you exhaling to your cat pose you're going to bring your elbows down towards your lap now your hands are on the head they're not pulling on it though right they're not pulling but you're letting the weight of the hands and the elbows with gravity give you just a little more stretch into the back of the neck we're going to inhale as we lift into cow pose exhale into cat pose inhale up into cow pose all right let's come back into cat pose think about tucking that chin let that head fall hands on that hip for a little extra weight one more breath here bring your hands down to your lap and lift very good did that feel okay all right so we're going to move to the back of our chair

back so I want you to have the back your back supported against the back of the chair so we're going to bring our knee into our chest okay so I've got my hands behind my thighs and I'm pulling that knee in and as you pull the knee in you're using the back of the chair to give you some support okay one more breath and let's bring that knee down and then we're going to go to the other side so we're squeezing so you should feel quite a little stretch here kind of where the hip and the leg

connect I feel it a little in my glute as well right a little bit into the hips feels good let's put that down we're going to do that one more time on each side before we add on so remember my in my classes you don't have to add on you can stay right here let's do one more on the other side okay so the add-on here is instead of leaning back and having the back supporting us we're going to move forward in our chair so now we have to use our abdominals right to provide that support because we don't have the chair

behind us so let's bring that knee in and squeeze I don't know if you notice but I'm lifting crown of the head to the ceiling right nice long spine bring it in squeeze it let's put it down we're going to do that one more time on each side so bring that knee in and squeeze okay so now the final piece of this is we're going to bring the knee in and squeeze and then we're going to bring it just a little bit across our body doesn't have to be a huge motion but I want you to feel a little more stretch

right here so all I'm doing is I'm bringing this knee across okay now what I'm going to do is I'm going to grab my leg with this hand and I'm going to open it hold that chair give yourself some support there so do you feel that inner thigh stretching right okay we're going to bring that knee in and we'll put that foot down okay we're going to go to the other side so let's start by just bringing the knee in lengthening nice and long through the spine so I'm not leaning back here right

I'm nice and long and if you're if you are sitting back with your back against the back of the chair that's fine I still want the crown of the head nice and long okay are we ready we're going to bring that leg across just a little bit of stretch here again it's a pretty subtle moon it's not huge then you're going to grab with this hand and you're going to open you can hold on to that chair make sure your abdominals stay tight through this we just had one more breath let's bring

that knee in and put that foot down can we do that one more time on each side let's do it bring it in and cross and open maybe you don't hold the chairs how does that feel come Center and put that foot down Let's go to the other side bring it in cross open Center and down all right very good work so now this is a gentle twist so I'm going to take my right hand and I'm going to just place it on the outside of that left knee do you see that nice long spine so anytime we're going to twist the spine whether we're forward

back side to side we want that spine to be super long before we do anything so let's take the hand here lengthen through the spine opposite hand to the chair pull this shoulder back and then we're just going to turn and look over that shoulder and we're going to Face Forward okay we're going to do that on the other side so this hand goes to the outer edge of that knee opposite hand back to the chair what do we do next lengthen through the spine right pull that shoulder back turn and look over that shoulder

and release okay so that's a great version of that series if you want a little bit more what we're going to do is we're going to take our left foot and we're going to cross it ankle to ankle now Did you notice I didn't move this leg stayed right where it was I just crossed ankle to ankle bring your hand to the outside of that knee opposite hand to the chair lengthen through the spine pull the shoulder back turn and look now we're going to face forward and we're going to go the other way so we're

going to take this hand on the outside of that knee opposite hand to the chair lengthen pull the shoulder back turn and look let's release that and then we're going to cross the other way the other ankles on top all right are we ready let's take this hand on the outside of that knee opposite hand to the chair lengthen and twist Face Forward opposite hand comes to this opposite knee other hand to the chair lengthen through the spine pull the shoulder back turn and look so just breathing here one more breath and face forward verygood how did that feel a little movement for that spine that feels okay so next we're going to do a seated forward fold and we're going to revolve it this is a very gentle version okay so we're going to move to the back of our chair so that the seat of the chair is between our legs okay so I know this can be a pretty big stretch for you so just take your time go ahead and give your legs a moment here to stretch into this particular position before we start okay so we're gonna have our hands right

here on the seat of our chair both Palms are down and all we're going to do is begin to let our hip and our heart fall forward okay so we're just letting that heart fall forward so this keeping your back flat so I'm thinking about looking out not down so look out towards me keep the back flat nice long spine so I'm lengthening through that spine kind of like thinking about head forward and seat back does that make sense all right let's tuck our chin and roll up okay can we do that again lengthen through the spine

let that heart begin to fall forward and Tuck the chin let's roll it up let's go ahead and bring our knees in and just take a break here for just a moment so what we're going to do now is the add-on for that forward fold is we're going to revolve it and all that means is we're just going to add a little twist okay A little rotation so just if it feels okay for you you're going to do the rotation if that doesn't feel okay for you then you're going to stay where you were all right are we

ready let's go ahead and open those legs back wide again make sure your seat is way back to the back of that chair hands are going to be right here on that chair Palms facing down we're going to begin to let that heart fall forward keeping the back flat okay so now all I'm going to do is I'm going to take my right hand and I'm going to move it to the center-right to the center and I'm going to take my left arm and I'm going to twist it up towards the ceiling so this is a very gentle

movement I want you to think about the action happening right at the ribs okay so my ribs rib cage is what's moving this arm is just kind of coming along for the ride I don't want the arm or the shoulder to initiate the movement I want the ribs to initiate the movement so again my arm is not that that far back at all right it's just kind of leaf lengthening up towards the ceiling super gentle here let's bring this hand back down and then we're going to go the other way okay are you feeling it super gentle

one more breath here all right let's go ahead and bring both hands down lift your heart bring those legs in and we're just going to do that one more time so I can't over-emphasize how important it is not to over-extend those shoulders so when we lift that arm the action happens at the ribs and the shoulder and the arm are just coming along for the right let's do it open those legs up make sure the hips are back are we ready hands on the chair to begin with let that heart fall forward now let's take our left hand and kind of

place it right in the center of the chair and we're going to let our right arm lengthen up towards the ceiling your rib cage is moving your ribs are stacking and then we're going to bring that hand we're going to replace the one on the chair and we're going to revolve it up and the other way are you feeling the stretch one more breath bring the hands back down to the chair lift I don't know about you but I was feeling my inner thighs stretching I was feeling the movement in the rib cage I was feeling

my back it's a nice nice gentle movement for the center of the body at least I thought it was all right so we're gonna move into our shavasana pose which is our relaxation pose so let's go ahead and sit back in our chair place your hands lightly on your thighs we're going to flip our palms up towards the ceiling take a deep breath in a full breath out let's take another deep breath in and as you exhale close your eyes exaggeration you wasted 30 minutes this morning so now the whole day is ruined

no, actually it's not you gave into temptation and ate a cinnamon roll so now you decide you'll never be able to lose weight but that thought is nothing but an extreme exaggeration it's helpful to recognize problems and mistakes so you can correct them and avoid them in the future yet exaggeration is not helpful at all yes perhaps you wasted some time early in the day however you have the rest of the day to make up for it instead of punishing yourself endlessly for a small slip take the opportunity to let it motivate

instead of exaggerating problems so far out of proportion that you give up do what's necessary to solve them get Beyond them make sure your thought process is working for you rather than against you see the problems and challenges realistically for what they are and enable yourself to successfully deal with them take a deep breath in and a full breath out open your eyes we're going to draw that right ear towards the right shoulder reach out with the right hand give the head a gentle tug as you press

that left hand down towards the floor release it drop your chin towards your chest reach up with your hands give the head a gentle tug release it drop your left ear towards your left shoulder reach up with the left hand give the head a gentle tug pressing that right hand down towards the floor release it look up just slightly open your mouth if you want to stretch your jaw bring your hands to your heart honoring one another we say namaste well done my fellow bottoms downies we've made it to the end of day three

DAY 4

Today is day four of our 28 day chair yoga journey together we're going to stay seated again today and we're going to add on a sun salutation so this is a series of poses that connects together into a sequence that warms up the body okay so we use it generally at the beginning of class to warm up and get the blood flowing now

let's get started so we're going to start by sitting up nice and tall and we're going to move forward in our chair so we're not leaning back now if you remember from day one how we start our practice focusing on the mind and the body and the breath so we're going to continue to do that and we'll start by grounding our feet to the floor okay so thinking about having both of your feet on the floor and also they're equally weighted so you don't feel like

you're moving your feet one way or the other everything is equally weighted and now the next thing we're going to do is ground those sits bones right so same idea where we have those pointy bones at the bottom of the pelvis that are on that chair and they're equally weighted so we're not leaning one way or the other okay all right we're gonna lift our heart up and we're going to lower our shoulders down out of our ears place your hands lightly on your thighs flip the Palms up towards the ceiling

now close your eyes if you wish and if you don't like closing your eyes just simply soften them connect to the breath and just simply breathe so this is our opportunity to connect into that breath so that body mind and breath and we're going to move that breath down into our diaphragm so as we inhale the belly will extend so we're moving it down into that belly breath we call it and then as you exhale you're going to pull your belly button in towards the spine pushing the air up and out of the

lungs let's do that again inhale and exhale let's do that one more time inhale exhale and just breathe normally bring your hands to your heart set your intentions for today's practice we have one more breath here all right let's bring our hands back down to our side our thighs and Open the Eyes ah all right we're just gonna simply look side to side so let's just take our gaze over that right shoulder to begin with now this is a gentle movement okay so we're not you know making it too intense we're going to look Center and then we're going to look the other way and then let's do that one more time all right we're looking Center we're going to look out to the right maybe take that gauge just a little further over that shoulder and look Center and then we're going to look the other way and let's look Center so what we're going to do now is we're going to bring our arms down by our side and we're going to shrug our shoulders up into our ears and then you're just simply going to let

them fall so you're letting gravity help let's shrug those shoulders up into the ears and let them fall one more time shrug the shoulders up into the ears and then just let them fall excellent work okay so now I'm going to take my left ear and I'm just going to let it fall towards my left shoulder okay so it's just kind of that ear to shoulder right there and that's all I want you to think about for right now just feel that stretch and then we're going to come up and we're going to go to the other side all

right so just a little next stretch here just gentle all right now come up so we're going to add one little thing to that and remember you don't ever have to add on to my class right ever ever okay so we're going to let that ear fall to the shoulder first and then I want you to just reach up with your hand now you're going to place it on the head but you're not going to pull and you're not going to tug you're just going to let the weight of that hand give you just a little extra stretch

now the final add-on is you're going to extend that opposite arm out so you're going to flex the wrist and push through the palm of the hand do you feel that just a little neck stretch here one more breath all right let's bring the hand down first opposite hand comes off of the head and lift that head up you may have to help it a little bit and you feel that Ah that's a good stretch okay let's go to the other side now we're going to let that ear fall towards the shoulder so we're just going to hang

out here for a moment so kind of get that natural Ranger motion first now I'm going to bring my hand up and place it lightly on the head I'm not pulling and I'm not tugging opposite arm is going to extend we're going to flex through the wrist push through the palm of the hand towards that side wall ah we have one more breath here let's bring that hand down let's take the hand off of the head bring that head up how's that feel okay very very good I'm just moving my head a little bit I don't know if you want to join me on that ah okay so we're going to move into our Mountain pose we've done this one before again it's a good warm-up pose so we're going to bring those hands to Heart okay now we're going to bring our arms down by our side and let's spread those fingers out very good how's that feel just a nice little stretch for those fingers okay come up to go go post Stars we're going to squeeze those shoulder blades back behind us so think about pulling the shoulders down and back alright so kind of a squeeze back there and now we're just going to lengthen those arms up towards the ceiling I don't know if you notice but I pulled my shoulders down right so we don't want those shoulders to come up we want to keep the shoulders down but we're lengthening the fingertips up towards the ceiling belly is tight we have one more breath here and let's bring those hands down to our lap okay we're moving right along now we're going to bring our hands to our heart now what I want you to think about is lifting up

through the spine okay so nice long crown of the head to the ceiling nice long spine we're opening up through the throat just a little bit here you feel that okay so we're going to first move into our cow pose thumbs to the back wall so I'm just opening up my chest do you feel that so pull that belly in keep the belly tight shoulders are down kind of squeezing the shoulder blades back behind you right thumbs to that back wall now we're going to move into our cat pose so I'm going to take my hands I'm

going to place them on my thighs elbows are wide pull your belly button to your spine tuck the chin and look at your belly so a nice rounded spine let the head fall feel the stretch in the back and in the back of the neck okay let's come back into cow pose again we're going to add the breath remember if you don't want to add the brushes breathe naturally it's fine but if you're with me we're going to inhale into cow pose and we're going to Exhale into cat's pose we're going to inhale into cow pose

and we're going to Exhale into cat's pose one more time inhale into cow pose and exhale into cat let's come back up into seated position and release I love that it kind of we begin to warm up that spine a little bit right getting a little a little blood flowing so we're going to do a seated twist and we're going to do it a couple of different ways and I'm going to let you pick and choose the version that you like the best so we're going to start with our feet on the floor knees are

forward we're going to take our right hand and we're going to place it on the outside of that left knee other hand is going to come to the chair back behind you okay now this is important I want you to pull this shoulder back then you're just going to turn and look over that shoulder so it's a gentle little twist here but your hand on the outside of that leg gives you a little bit of Leverage to where you can add a little additional twist in here if that feels okay for you let's go ahead and face forward and we're going to go to the other side okay so my left hand is on the outside of the right knee opposite hand to the chair lengthen through the spine pull the shoulder back turn and look so we're hanging out here and we're breathing alright one more breath here and we're gonna Face Forward okay so those are that's a great version and if you like that one you're going to stick with it now if you want to add on with me we're going to leave this right leg where it is and we're going to take our left

ankle and we're going to cross it at the ankle so it's an ankle to ankle but I didn't bring this leg in I left it out did you see that okay right hand to the outside of that knee opposite hand to the chair don't forget to lengthen through the spine first pull that left shoulder back turn and look so it's a little different stretch a little different twist here I want the action happening right at the rib cage go ahead and face forward and let's go ahead and release that and we're going to go to the other side okay

so we're going to cross that ankle to ankle hand to the outside of the knee opposite hand back to the chair lengthen through the spine pull the shoulder back turn and look and then just hang out and breathe here make sure those shoulders are staying down trying to get the action to happen right at the ribs one more breath and face forward and release okay so the final piece of this only if you want you've got two other really good versions but if you want it we're going to cross leg over leg so it's kind of knee on top

of me okay all right are we ready we're going to take our right hand we're going to place it on the inside of that leg opposite hand back we're going to lengthen through the spine pull the shoulder back turn and look so it just changes the Dynamics doesn't it knees stay forward hips stay forward the twist is happening at the ribs one more breath Face Forward okay let's unravel that and then we're going to go straight to that other side so we're going to take the other leg on top this hand is going to go on the

inside opposite hand to the chair don't forget the lengthen through the spine pull the shoulder back turn and look we're breathing we're not holding our breath holding the posture but not the breath one more breath here face forward and release okay very good we feel good that little movement going right there through that that rib cage I love that love those little twists super gentle though right we're always very gentle with our twisting okay so we're gonna move into I promised you that sun

salutation so we're going to move into that now and I'm going to take it very slow and we're going to do piece by piece okay so and and then we'll then what we'll do is we'll move through it several more times with a little more fluidity all right okay so bring your hands to your heart we're going to start here all right now we're going to make a big circle so Palms are going to face up all right so we're going to come all the way up Palms are going to be together above you so this is an

extended Mountain pose right belly's tight we're going to bring our hands to Heart now I'm going to bring my hands back up back to that extended mountain and I'm going to make that big circle around and I'm going to bring my hands to my heart okay we're gonna do that again so if you'll notice we've got quite a bit of movement in those shoulders so if that's bothering your shoulders you're going to keep your elbows bent so maybe let I'll show you here so let's do it again and

I'm going to do it with bent elbows you see how I'm just keeping my elbows bent so that's going to take some of that pressure off of those shoulders so if you've got shoulder issues bring your hands to heart and then we're going to come up and we're going to make that circle around and we're going to bring our hands to heart all right are we ready let's do it again here we go inhale let's add that breath inhale up we go exhale hands to Heart do that again ml up exhale big circle around bring your

hands to your heart we're gonna do that one more time before we add on ready big circle up we go extended Mountain I'm watching my hands with my gaze bring your hands to Heart did you notice that inhale up we go follow that gate your hands with your gaze big circle around and bring your hands to your heart okay let's bring our hands down and take just a moment you feeling alright with that you notice that that alternative here that little variation with the bent elbow so remember that one is fine

so now the next pose we're going to add is a forward salute with airplane arms now if you do matte yoga this is kind of what we the variation we use instead of halfway lift okay so it's the same idea you're still getting that lengthening through the spine so here let's all do it together to begin with so I'm going to bring my arms back by my side this is those airplane arms I call it right so they're back by the side my fingertips are pointing down where the floor and the and the wall meet okay and I'm

stretching then I want my head to go forward kind of where the ceiling and the wall meet right so I'm strengthening I'm lengthening through my spine super long through the spine you just kind of see what I'm doing there all right let's bring our hands to Heart we're going to add that in let's do it big circle inhale up we Mountain pose bring your hands to Heart let's go back to that mountain pose now we're going to dive It Forward belly button to spine and we're going to come to that forward salute

with our plane arms stretch you feel that nice long spine one more breath bring your hands to your heart let's do that again big circle up we go inhale exhale hands to Heart we're going to go back to that extended Mountain we're going to Swan Dive forward and we're going to come into that forward salute airplane arms and we're stretching through that spine let's bring our hands to heart and do it again before we add on up we go exhale hands to Heart can you add that diaphragmatic breath

inhale belly breath exhale dive it forward stretch it out and then just breathe naturally here one more breath bring your hands to your heart okay so the last thing we're going to add in to our sun salutation is a forward fold now we're going to do our forward fold today with support and what I mean by that is I'm going to put the forearms on my thighs and I'm going to let my heart fall forward so I'm supported right so I've got my arms here on my legs I've got full support and I can let my heart

fall forward there's that back stretching do you feel that I mean it's it seems like such a simple movement and yet I really feel my back stretching and you can let that heart fall a little bit further if you want because you've got that support okay does that make sense now to get out of this what I'd like for you to do is tuck your chin and roll up okay let's do that one more time let's come into that forward fold let that heart fall forward all right you feel the stretch I do okay and now to get out of it we're going to

tuck our chin and we're going to roll it up let's bring our hands to our heart are we ready full thing here we go big circle up inhale exhale bring your hands to Heart let's come back up to that extended Mountain dive it forward forward salute airplane arms stretch stretch stretch are we ready forward fold and how to prepare exhale as we come forward you notice that I'm looking out I'm not looking down at the floor I'm looking out I'm keeping my back flat I'm feeling that stretch

one more breath tuck the chin roll it up bring your hands to your heart are we ready big circle inhale up we go exhale hands to Heart big circle up dive it forward forward salute airplane arms stretch it out forward fold use that breath if you wish let that heart fall a little bit further tuck the chin roll it up this is our last time make it get a big circle up we go and bring those hands to heart doesn't it feel good up we go dive it forward forward salute airplane arms stretch let's do that supported forward fold let that heart

fall forward are we ready tuck the chin roll it up and release oh my goodness that was so good you guys it feels so good I love that when we're moving we're getting the blood flowing we're getting a little a little heat I don't know about you but you're beginning to feel a little heat building up in the body so it's excellent work all right we're going to move into our shavasana pose now so we're gonna go ahead and sit back in our chair let's place our hands lightly on our

thighs flip those Palms up let's take a deep breath in and a full breath out take a deep breath in and on this exhalation close your eyes or soften the eyes quality time give quality time to yourself give quality time to others spend time doing what helps you feel good about yourself about the people around you about the world you live in who what improves your health your relationships your understanding your sense of well-being seek out areas of your daily life where you can add your own unique flavor of

Excellence devote time thought and effort to increase the amount of joy in your world the moment you focus on quality will continue to bring benefits long after those moments have passed the joys you add to the experience of Life can never be taken away each day you have a finite amount of time available make it your mission to spend that time enhancing enjoying and sharing life's best qualities enable life to more fully experience its own richness with your attitude your outlook and your actions make as much of your time as you

can into quality time take a deep breath in a full breath out open your eyes we're going to drop our right ear towards our right shoulder you jump with the right hand give the head just the gentlest of tugs just so so gentle press that left hand down towards the floor god it feels so good and let's release it let's drop our chin towards our chest we're going to reach up with our hands again just giving that head a super gentle tongue and release it drop your left ear towards your left shoulder reach up with the left hand now giving

that head the scent just a gentle tug right hand extends out if that feels okay and release now we're going to look up just slightly if you want to open your mouth to stretch that jaw go for it bring your hands to your heart honoring one another we say namaste ah very well done my fellow bottoms and downings to the end of day four would you not agree that the hardest part is just getting to your chair once you're here isn't it fun isn't it lovely please keep showing up

DAY 5

So today is day five of our 28 day chair yoga Journey we're going to stay seated again today and we're going to add on some additional poses for the legs we'll do a crescent lunge and a pyramid pose now

let's get started so we're going to start moving forward in our chair all right we're sitting up nice and Tall we're not leaning back and remember as we connect our body and mind and breath let's Place both of our feet on the floor and we're going to ground each foot to the Earth to the Earth and now we're going to ground our sits bones okay so we're feeling like we're on the chair and everything is equally weighted let's lift our heart take those shoulders and move them down out of the ears place your hands lightly on your thighs flip the Palms facing up

close your eyes or soften the eyes and connect to your heart center now just notice your breath your natural inhalation and exhalation and with every breath see if you can feel like your spine is a little bit longer so as we think about that spine just remember right it holds us up pretty important so we want to keep that spine nice and long let's go ahead and deepen that breath so inhale just a little more deeply lengthening through the spine and exhale a little more completely let's do that again inhale

one more time inhale and exhale bring your hands to your heart and set your intentions for today's practice focusing in on what you want to accomplish one more breath here let's bring our hands down to our thighs we'll open our eyes We're Gonna Roll those shoulders so it's a little exaggerated shoulder roll here alright so it's kind of a thinking about forward and up and back and down and let's reverse that now let's go back and up and forward and down maybe do that one more time

still okay and release that should feel really really good so we're gonna move into an extended Mountain so we're going to take our hands towards the ceiling now as you do that I want you to really concentrate on keeping the shoulders down I want you to think about pulling your belly button into the spine so we're activating our abdominals right belly tight shoulders are down fingertips up towards the ceiling seems like a simple pose doesn't it extended Mountain but it's a very active pose as long as you're doing it with intention all right let's bring those hands down and take just a moment so we're going to be adding one thing on here next and remember you don't have to add on you can stay right where we were but if it's okay with you we're going to bring our hands back up now put the Palms together interlace your fingers but the pointer finger is towards the ceiling and I don't know if you've noticed but I've got to Bent my elbows a little bit okay so I'm not here right I'm pulling those shoulders down and

when I pull the shoulders down the elbows Bend just a little bit my abdominals are tight here all right really think about pulling your belly in now we're going to lean our Mountain now as you lean your Mountain what I want you to really focus in on is keeping this hip down right so you're going to feel two distinct stretches you'll feel a stretch from your hip tip this I call the pelvis here the hip tip to the armpit and then you'll feel the armpit out the pinky finger or maybe out the pointer finger since we're kind of

pointing that do you feel those two distinct stretches okay we're going to bring our hands to the ceiling let's pull the shoulders down one more time pull the belly in and then we're going to lean the other way do you feel that so very distinct feeling stretches keeping that hip down feeling the hip tip to the armpit armpit out the fingers I feel it very distinct stretches let's bring those hands back up we're going to bring the hands back down and I'm going to do a shoulder roll here I don't know if you

want to join me it just feels good right when I've had my hands up in the air like that for a while okay we're going to add one more thing into our extended mountain and that's going to be a little twist it's a very very subtle movement okay so don't feel like oh my gosh we're gonna be it's not a big one so let's go ahead and come back into that extended Mountain all right you notice how pull my shoulders down let's put the Palms together interlace your fingers and then extend your pointer finger to the

ceiling okay let's let's go ahead and lean to the left first this time all right now from here all you're going to do is you're just going to turn and look up at the ceiling it's pretty small but you'll feel it right right at the ribs that's where I feel it that's where I want you to feel it all right let's take the twist out and then we're going to come up and we're going straight to the other side let's do it let's start with our leaning Mountain first get this stretch feel those two distinct stretches now we're going to twist and look up at the ceiling belly is tight here we're protecting that low back just one more breath take the twist out bring the hands back up to the ceiling and bring the hands down to your lap how did that feel oh boy a little bit of movement right here at those at those ribs right okay we've done cat and cow now we're going to move into our cat and cow poses so let's take our thumbs to the back wall again for our cow pose you know what I could have started with that

open throat but just think about opening the throat here and then let's come down into that cat pose hands to those thighs elbows wide don't forget tuck the chin let that head fall look at your belly let's do that again and add the breath inhale up into our cow pose exhale round down into that cat pose let's do that again inhale come up into cow exhale come down into cat one more time inhale up into cow exhale down into cap and release do you remember yesterday we did that sun salutation we're gonna do it again

bring your hands to your heart ready here we go big circle up we go Mountain pose bring your hands to Heart we're going to inhale to prepare as we come up exhale we're going to move into that Swan dog belly button to spine you've got it stretch it out you feel that stretch one more breath bring your hands to your heart let's do that one more time before we add on big old Circle up we go bring your hands to your heart let's come back up to Extended Mountain dive It Forward into that forward salute

airplane arm stretch oh yeah and bring your hands to heart all right we're going to add that supported forward fold big go Circle up we go inhale exhale hands to heart you feeling it up we don't Mountain pose die forward Swan die forward salute airplane arms okay let's add that forward fold let's do it supported Palms are facing up forearms are on the thighs let that heart fall forward remember we're keeping the back flat so we're looking out not down okay keep that back flat can you let that heart

fall any further you're still supported you've got your arms on those thighs to protect it let's tuck the chin and roll it up and back we go to hands to heart now we're going to do that again but let's let me I'll say one thing here you know what what's happening in your body right and if that's supported forward fold if going that far forward doesn't work for you then maybe you stay right here it's okay I want you to listen to your body and what's happening to you but I'm just giving you some Alternatives right so that everybody can feel like they're getting getting um you know being successful and feeling like they're getting some some work and some stretch okay we're going to do that again we're going to do it a couple more times without stopping all right hands to Heart let's add that breath inhale up we go follow your hands with your gaze bring your hands to heart there's your exhale we're going to come back up into that inhale Mountain pose and it come

forward into that forward salute airplane arms we're going to come to that forward fold supported let that heart fall forward tuck the chin and roll it up and bring your hands to your heart let's do that again big circle up we go are you feeling like the blood flowing I know right we'll get that blood flowing up we go and that's your inhale die forward into that forward salute airplane arms we're stretching forward fold we got this right let that heart fall forward ready tuck the chin and roll it up hands

to Heart last time through beat a circle there's your inhale hands to heart is your exhale back up we go we're going to dive forward into that forward salute airplane arms and we're stretching we're going to come to that forward fold we know what we're doing don't we this one's so good tuck the chin and roll it up ha all right man we feel like we're moving now that is great okay so I promised you a couple of leg poses so we're going to move into the first one is called Crescent lunge so what I'm

going to do is I'm going to take my right knee and I'm going to open it now the very first thing I want you to feel is an inner thigh stretch and a pretty significant one isn't it so here's the thing this knee this one that's facing me needs to stay open okay so I want that knee to feel like it's open so we're not letting that knee fold in and I want you to feel that stretch first I know it's a pretty significant stretch okay so now we're going to let this knee fall down towards the floor and I'm going to

turn you see I'm kind of turning in my chair so now this leg is facing the wall here this knee is straight down towards the floor hold that chair or you can hold your thigh right just hold on so feel like you're stable okay so I'm just hanging out here and I'm breathing do you feel that stretch right yeah I feel it too so we're hanging out here and we're breathing we've got one more breath now we're going to come back up and face forward okay so we're gonna uh add that that pyramid pose next and we're going to do it on the same side and then we'll do both poses on the other side okay and then we're going to repeat it a couple of times so let's add that pyramid pose now because I kind of like we've just stretched the front side of the leg now we're going to stretch the back side of that same leg so extend your leg out in front of you the same one that was just the knee was down towards the mat right you feel that same leg extend nice and long through the spine and just letting your heart fall

forward so I'm looking out not down okay so look out look out look out keep the back flat belly is tight oh yeah we have one more breath let's tuck our chin and roll it up and we're going to bend that knee and put that foot on the floor okay so I'm just kind of we're going through it to begin with and then we're going to do it a few more times but let's do the other side first so we're going to take that left knee and open and again we're just taking a moment here to feel the inner thigh stretch all

right so make sure this knee is angling towards me and make sure this knee is towards that other wall okay so we're just we're just hanging here for a moment okay now we're going to let that right knee fall down towards the floor okay so just let that knee fall straight down hang hands can be on this thigh hands can be on the chair you feel it right okay just one more breath now face forward and we're going to move into pyramid pose same leg right leg toes to the ceiling lengthen through the spine holding on to

that fellow's thighs and let that heart fall forward so now we're getting the back side of that leg so the knee stays straight we don't we have a micro Bend of the knee but we don't want to bend this knee and I'm looking out not down my back is flat one more breath and roll it up okay so we're gonna do that again here we go right knee opens left knee Falls towards the mat now if you want a little bit more instead of this knee falling straight down to the mat what I'm going to do is

I'm up on my back toes and I'm going to press that leg back just a little bit oh yeah how's that feel so we're stretching the front side of this leg right here so quadricep and hip flexor should feel super good let's bend the knee relax it and then it's going to do that one more time okay let's face forward now we're going to move into pyramid pose we're going to extend that leg out toes to the ceiling lengthen through the spine let the heart fall forward there's your hamstring

stretch you feel it tuck the chin and roll it up we're gonna do that one more time nice long spine let that heart pop forward feels so good and Tuck that chin and roll it up let's do the other side here we go open you got it let this knee fall down towards the floor so let's start with the knee straight down just get that feeling first hanging onto the thighs or to the chair okay now if you want a little bit more I'm just pushing my foot back behind me my leg is long I'm up on those back toes

let's release it and we're going to stretch it one more time back in the kneecap kind of moves up towards the ceiling super gentle here though right we don't ever do anything drastic it's just gentle and face forward okay ready for a pyramid pose again extend that leg out in front of you toes to the ceiling we're going to lengthen nice and long through the spine I'm going to put my hands on my thighs and I'll let that heart fall forward ah we can add that breath if you want let's roll it up we're going to inhale

to prepare exhale down we go one more breath and roll it up excellent work okay let's go ahead and move back in our chair and get ready for our savasana pose our relaxation pose so we're gonna have our hands in our lap flip those Palms up to the ceiling take a deep breath in and a full breath out take a deep breath in and on this exhalation close your eyes or soften your eyes fulfill the potential give yourself credit for how far you've come

then challenge yourself to build on it life has not been perfect yet you've successfully navigated your way to today now you can use your skills in tention and persistence to move forward recognize that you've established some positive momentum consider what you can do to grow that momentum put it to purposeful use you have gained strength from everything you've been through what good things can you now do to exercise that strength through your life experiences you've earned wisdom and gained a unique

perspective you're better positioned than ever before to act with purpose passion Effectiveness and understanding your past has prepared you for the challenges of the future rise up meet those challenges and fulfill the potential that's been accumulating throughout your whole life a deep breath in and a full breath out drop your right ear towards your right shoulder reach up with the right hand give the head a gentle tug as you press that left hand down towards the floor release her drop your chin towards your chest

reach up with the hands give the head a gentle tug release it drop your left ear towards your left shoulder reach up with the left hand give the head a gentle tug pressing that right hand down towards the floor release it look up just slightly open your mouth if you want to stretch your jaw bring your hands to your heart honoring one another we say namaste ah very well done

DAY 6

let's get started so we're going to move forward in our chair we're not leaning back okay and we're going to take a moment to connect our body and our mind and our breath so let's put both of our feet on the floor thinking about grounding those feet we have equal weight in both feet they're not pronated they're not supinated they're both equally weighted on the on the floor and the same thing with our sits bones we have those pointy bones that we sit on and we want to have them on the chair and equally weighted okay so let's lift our heart up consciously think about taking those shoulders down out of the ears okay so

think about it pulling them down place your hands on the thighs flip those Palms up towards the ceiling close your eyes or soften the Gaze and breathe just thinking about with every inhalation we extend through the spine and release take a deep breath in extending through that spine and exhale we're going to move that breath down into our diaphragm so as we inhale the breath moves out of our shoulders and chests and moves down into that belly we're filling those lungs from the bottom up so let's take a deep breath ex

a diaphragmatic breath and then as we exhale we actively pull the belly button in towards the spine and push the air up and out of the lung so it's a very active breath do that a couple more times and breathe normally bring your hands to your heart set your intentions for today's practice focusing in on what you want to accomplish just one more breath here bring your hands back down to your thighs and open your eyes We're Gonna Roll those shoulders again today it just feels good right so it's kind of a forward and an up and a back

and a Down I call it the super exaggerated shoulder roll so I want you to really feel each area right each Direction and then we're going to reverse it so try to really bring them forward and let them come down squeeze them behind up we go let's do that again forward and down and squeeze behind and up and release okay so we're going to do our cat and cow for our cow pose let's grab the back of the chair today squeezing the shoulder blades behind you and lifting up so it's kind of an openness through the throat feeling a

brightness in the chest opening up through that heart and then we're going to come down into our cat pose hands to thighs elbows wide tuck the chin and look down at your belly button let's lift up grab the back of the chair squeeze those shoulder blades back behind you lifting up looking up feeling that openness in the throat and in the heart and then round down into that cat pose make sure you're letting the head fall and let's do that one more time and we're lifting that we're doing a

little slower today aren't we we're not actually adding that breath because we're doing it so slowly the breath would be kind of hard so just breathe naturally and then let's come down into that cat pose again and release okay very good so we're going to move into extended Mountain we're going to take our hands up to the ceiling shoulders are down now you're going to take your right hand to the chair and I want you to extend that left hand like you're trying to touch the ceiling and then we're going

to lean okay that feels good now I want you to take your hand up to the ceiling and you're going to turn and look up okay let's lean that mountain again and then we're going to take our hand to the ceiling and we're going to turn and look up now your right hand is on the chair for support okay let's lean one more time oh that feels good hand to the ceiling turn and look up and then we're going to bring that hand down okay let's do the other side extending that mountain nice and long

okay now the left hand is going to come to the chair extend that right hand up towards the ceiling but shoulders stay down belly is tight okay are we ready let's learn that mountain feel that stretch on the side waist take your hand to the ceiling we're going to turn and we're going to look up just a little twist here and then we're going to lean our Mountain again hand to the ceiling turn and look up and we're gonna do that one more time lean that mountain take the hand up towards the ceiling

turn and look up and release all right very very good okay we've done our sun salutations now for a couple of days in a row so we're gonna do it again bring those hands to Heart are we ready we're going to make our big circle up we go all the way to Mountain pose and we're going to bring our hands to our heart now we're going to take our hands to the ceiling and we're going to make a big circle around and we're going to bring our hands back to our heart and we're going to go all

the way back up into a mountain pose extended Mountain interlace your fingers Point your fingers to the ceiling we're going to lean that mountain I just threw that in didn't I let's come up and we're going to lean that mountain the other way hello and we're going to come up and we're just going to bring those arms around and we're going to bring our hands to our heart let's do that again big circle up we go Mountain pose hands to heart this time we're going to extend our mountain and we're

going to come into that Swan Dive let's do it airplane arms remember stretching those fingers back towards the where the wall and the floor meet stretching our head where the ceiling in the wall meet we're feeling that stretch and we're going to bring our hands to our heart let's do that again before we add on big circle up extended Mountain bring your hands to Heart let's come back up and we're going to dive forward into that forward salute we got those airplane arms again we're stretching

let's move into that forward fold let's support it let that heart fall forward I promise you later on we're going to get to a more more deep forward fold we're going to tuck our chin and roll up but for right now we're going to stay with this supported version here we go up we go and we're going to bring our hands to Heart we're going to come back up into that mountain pose and we're going to dive it forward forward salute our plane arms stretch it out let's do that supported forward fold let that heart

fall forward all right tuck that chin and roll it up let's add the breath inhale up we go exhale hands to Heart inhale up we go exhale dive it forward inhale prepare exhale forward fold tuck the chin and roll it up last time bring your hands to Heart they go Circle up we go bring your hands to Heart we're coming back up into that mountain pose extended Mountain forward salute airplane arms stretch forward fold we got this we know what we're doing and Tuck that chin and roll it up a lot of movement in that one isn't

there all right so we're going to move into a half lord of the fish's pose so I actually we remember from yesterday we did this first stretch first piece of it so we're going to take this right knee and open okay so this is the beginning part of our half lord of the fish's pose now this knee has got to stay forward okay so it's going to want to bend in I'm just telling you already I know what's going to happen don't let that happen all right we're going to keep that knee open make that inner

thigh stretch and work now you're going to take your left hand see how I'm opening it up now I'm going to bring that arm all the way across my body and I'm going to grab my chair you see what's happening there I've got my chair now I'm going to lengthen through the spine and I'm going to turn and I'm going to look over the back of my chair okay so you're not looking at me now you're looking over the back of your chair it's okay I haven't gone anywhere I'm still here

let's release the arms leave the legs where they are and we're going to do that again all right we're going to bring that arm all the way across our body we're going to grab our chair lengthen through the spine turn and look over the back of your chair and breathe now everybody I want you to peek at that left knee is it folding in go ahead and look at it it's folding in don't let it open it up one more breath and release so we're going to move straight into that Crescent lunge remember we did Crescent

lunge yesterday we're going to take this knee and we're going to drop it down maybe we push our foot back a little bit right we're up on those back toes we're facing forward and then we're going to let that knee fall down towards the floor and then we're going to push the back of the kneecap up towards the ceiling a little bit if that feels okay for you one more breath and we're going to face forward that same leg we're going to extend it out in front of us toes to the ceiling we're going to lengthen and

hinge into our pyramid pose and Tuck the chin and roll it up and we're going to do that again this is a little sequence I really like half lord of the fishes to Crescent lunge to Pyramid pose and roll it up we're going to go to the other side okay so now we're going to take our left knee and we're going to open it nice and wide this knee stays open okay are we ready right arm opens up we're going to breathe across the body grab the chair lift the crown of the head to the ceiling turn and look over

the back of your chair everybody turn and peek at that knee is it folding in I know it wants to you know if it really is hard you can heel toe your foot in a little bit I would rather you have the knee and the ankle in alignment and have the foot in a little bit then have the foot out in the knee folding in okay so does that make sense all right let's open and we're gonna do that again bringing across the body grab that chair lift the crown of the head to the ceiling turn and look over the back of your chair and breathe

we just have one more breath all right let's release that moving into Crescent lunge here we go let that knee fall down towards the floor push that foot back behind you hold on to that chair lift that heart that feel good it should feel really good stretching right here right let's release it and we're gonna do that one more time ah and we're gonna face forward and we're going to extend that leg out in front of us toes to the ceiling lengthen and hinge keep that back flat you got it tuck the

chin and roll it up extend nice and long and let that heart fall forward oh yeah and Tuck that chin and roll it up okay so we're going to do that one more time and we're just going to kind of flow through it right it's a little bit of a vinyasa flow if you will okay and all that means is that we're just connecting a few poses together there's nothing fancy about that okay so we're going to take that knee we're going to open it we're going to bring that arm and open it and come across the body grab the

chair lift the crown ahead turn and look over the back of your chair and let's do that again open breathe across the bottom lift and twist and release knee falls down towards the floor push the foot back we're going to do one little ad on here okay lifting up through the heart feeling that stretch let's bring our arms to to go post arms or goddess arms so I'm lifting up through the heart chin is open I'm looking at kind of where the ceiling and the wall meet let's release that and we're going to do

that one more time let's do it oh yeah one more breath and release Face Forward we're gonna do our pyramid pose now we've done static versions previously we're going to add a little Dynamic stretch here so lengthen through the spine we're going to bring the hands up then we're going to bring them out and we're going to bring them down towards our foot oh yeah and then roll it up inhale exhale out and down one more time coming up inhale exhale out and down excellent work bend that knee put that

foot on the floor straight to the other side here we go open it up bring that arm across grab that chair lift through the crown of the head towards the ceiling turn and look over the back of the chair leave that knee open open it up let's do that again bring that hand across the the to the chair extend through the spine turn and look over the back of your chair and release let this knee fall down towards the floor Crescent lunge press that foot back we got it don't we lift that heart up let's release it are we ready to add the

arms let's press this back of the kneecap up come up go post arms looking up slightly just a little stretch we're gonna release it let's do that one more time squeezing the shoulder blades back behind you opening up through the throat one more breath and release Turn To Face Forward pyramid pose extend that right leg out are we ready inhale extend the hands to the ceiling exhale hands come out towards the wall in front of you and then down towards the floor band up come up into seated extend the arms inhale exhale out

and down let's do that one more time up we go inhale extend exhale out and down and up we go let that feel and a lot of movement today didn't we yeah so we weren't really holding our poses very long today we were moving through okay that's very good so we're going to move into our shavasana pose so now we can lean back I know doesn't that feel good we work so hard flip those ponds up towards the ceiling close the eyes and just breathe give Beauty give life Beauty make something beautiful do something

beautiful experience and share something beautiful life and Beauty intertwined to the benefit of both Beauty carries life and purpose and inspiration forward and life makes beauty possible in the service of beauty you learn valuable skills in the experience of beauty you discover important truths about who you are in your actions your words your attitude be beautiful live in a way that adds unique beauty to the experience of the people you encounter your efforts and commitments are about more than just getting by

you have the opportunity and the ability to contribute Beauty to the world notice the beauty appreciate the beauty feel the beauty and expand on the beauty that is such a significant part of life let's take a deep breath in and a full breath out drop your right ear towards your right shoulder reach up with the right hand give the head a gentle tug as you press that left hand down towards the floor release it drop your chin towards your chest reach up with your hands give the head a gentle tug release it

drop your left ear towards your left shoulder reach up with the left hand give the head a gentle tug as you press that right hand down towards the floor release it look up just slightly open your mouth if you want to stretch your jaw bring your hands to your heart honoring one another we say namaste so much so good very well done

DAY 7

let's get started so we're going to sit up nice and tall in our chair we're not leaning back nice long spine shoulders are down out of the ears take a moment to ground those feet to the Earth and your sits bones to the chair let's lift our heart and lower shoulder shoulder take your hands lightly on the thighs lift the Palms up close your eyes and connect to your breath we're going to elongate that breath now inhaling a little more deeply exhaling a little more completely we're going to move into that diaphragmatic breath as we inhale we're going to fill those

lungs from the bottom up our belly will extend and then as we exhale we're going to pull our belly button towards our spine and push the air up and out of the lungs so do that a couple of times and breathe normally we're going to continue with our diaphragmatic breath we're going to inhale to four counts and exhale to five counts it'll be something like this inhale two three four exhale two three four five inhale two three four exhale two three four five and breathe normally bring your hands to your heart set your

intentions for today's practice one more breath here bring your hands back down to your thighs and open your eyes so we're going to start our relaxation series with alternate nostril breathing now this particular breathing technique is where we're going to breathe in one nostril and out the other and the intention here is to balance your energy and quiet the mind so what we're going to do is we're going to inhale to begin and then we're going to take our thumb and place it right up against our nostril right so let's

inhale and then we're going to push our thumb on our nostril and we're going to Exhale now with your finger you're going to close off the other nostril and inhale and then you're going to close and exhale one more time inhale and exhale now take just a moment here we're going to take that really slow and steady okay so we don't want to do it too quickly we don't want to get dizzy so if it begins to make you dizzy then just breathe normally it's okay and the final thing see if you can make that

exhalation longer than the inhalation let's switch hands just for the fun of it all right so we're going to inhale my thumb is going to go up against that nostril and let's exhale finger to the nostril inhale thumb exhale finger inhale and exhale and release do you feel like it's kind of quieted your mind right I just love that very

very good okay so what we're going to do next is we're going to have our hands back behind our back excuse me back behind our back okay so we're going to squeeze our shoulder

blades back just a little bit you don't have to like make it tremendous with just a little squeeze here and my thumbs or my Knuckles are going down towards the chair okay so hands behind my back Knuckles to chair squeeze and we're going to make little circles with our nose okay so it's just a little circle and then we're going to begin to make that Circle a little bigger and then we're going to make the circle a little bit bigger and now it's a pretty big circle let's stop and we're going to reverse it

we're going to start big and then we're going to begin to tighten up that coil then we're going to make it a little bit tighter and a little bit smaller and a tiny little circle and release that okay very good so the next thing is a is a chin to chest neck stretch so we'll start by stacking our palms together in our lap so I have one Palm on top of the other and they're just resting in my lap now I want you to extend your thumbs okay we're going to bring our hands up and then we're going to bring them back

behind our head so our hands are going to be right behind our head and they're it's kind of cradling our head now with those extended thumbs you're going to give yourself a little massage on the neck do you feel that right just a little massage there okay now inhale we're going to extend the chin up towards the ceiling bring the front of those ribs in pull the belly in now we're not initiating the movement with the back but we're initiating the movement with the neck we're going to

bring those elbows forward and then down and exhale as we let those elbows come down towards the chair so you're not pulling on the head you're letting gravity do the work here let's take our hands off of the head and let's lift that head up okay so how did that feel did that feel okay let's just move around just a little bit okay we're going to do that again we kind of know what we're doing now right okay hands are going to stack the one Palm on top of the other in our lap extend the thumbs long

bring those hands up and you're going to bring your hands back behind your head elbows are nice and wide now your extended thumbs you're going to give yourself just a little massage there okay now lifting up through the chin right so bring those ribs in here we go inhale elbows come up towards the ceiling and then exhale we're going to bring those elbows down towards the mat don't pull on the head just let gravity do the work here and then we're just going to take a few breaths just one more breath release the hands

and lift the head up and move around just a little bit we're going to do that one more time because I like it it feels really good ready here we go stack those Palms extend those thumbs up we go hands behind the head give yourself a little massage with those extended thumbs lifting up inhale to prepare exhale elbows to the ceiling and down we go remember don't pull on the head just let gravity do the work here we initiate that movement with the neck not the back we have one more breath we're going to

release our hands down and roll it up all that feels pretty good to me maybe you move that neck around just a little bit the next thing are elbow circles so we're going to take our hands and we're going to place them on our shoulders and then we're going to lift those elbows up and they're going to kiss each other now we're going to take those elbows up towards the ceiling stretching like elbow up and then we're going to bring the elbows back squeezing back behind and then we're going to let the elbows

fall towards the floor now the weight of the elbow so you're just kind of holding on here and the weight of those elbows is going to give you a little stretch for the top of those shoulders let's not our head units let's shake our head no and not our head yes all right now we're going to reverse that okay so hands are still here on the thigh on the shoulders we're going to bring those elbows back squeeze oh yeah and up we go bring them forward kiss and down and do a little head knot oh yeah and a

head shake and a head knob we're gonna do that one more time all right are we ready up we go kiss elbows up to the ceiling I want you to really feel the stretch elbows up up up up up now we're going to bring them back behind us kind of so squeezing the shoulder blades back behind now let those elbows fall towards the floor so holding on to those shoulders let's do a head knot I like it and a shake and a knot okay we gotta go the other way are we ready up we go back squeeze elbows up to the ceiling stretch

down they go kiss elbows towards the floor and release ah that feels so good to me that's a really really good one too okay so now we're going to do a little bit for the scalings I don't know about you but my scalings are always so tight these muscles right here on the side of the neck right so what I'm going to do is I'm going to take my right hand and I'm going to place it on the opposite collarbone now what you're going to do is you're I want to move my hair so you can see so

my hand is above that collarbone and I want you to pin those muscles okay so I'm kind of pushing in just a little bit and I'm going to try to hold those muscles in place and then I'm going to look down over this shoulder and down now I'm going to look Center and then I'm going to look up and I'm going to look Center let's do that again look down and center and look up and release did you feel that let's do the other side so I'm going to put my hand just run above the collarbone right I'm gonna push in just

gently kind of hold those muscles we call that pinning pinning those muscles okay now I'm going to look over this shoulder okay I already feel it I don't know about you but maybe this side's tighter than the other I don't know okay now look down yeah baby ambulance Center and look up and look Center let's do that one more time Loop down look Center and look up and center and release that feels really good to me so kind of move around a little bit if you want to okay so we're going to interlace our fingers

and we're going to press those Palms out now we're going to have those hands up towards the ceiling I'm about to sneeze so just ah it went away all right we're going to lean I just like all of a sudden a little distracted there with my nose itching and needing to sneeze and therefore we go and then we're going to lean the other way and up we go now I want you to bring those hands back down into your lap now I want you to notice which pinky fingers on bottom and you're going to interlace your

fingers the other way and it feels very weird I know are we ready here we go Palms out oh yeah and up and lean and up and lean and up and release and shake it out just a little bit okay so now interlace your fingers your normal way and this one is we call this ride the wave and it's a little funky so just do whatever feels good for you but basically what I'm going to do is I'm going to bend this wrist you see how now this arm is parallel to the mat I've got my wrist bent and then this arm is straight and then I'm going to do the

other right so it's just kind of a rotting the wave we're just stretching into those wrists a little bit don't worry too much about how you're doing it it doesn't matter and then let's reverse that direction should feel good let's do one more beautiful okay let's release that and shake it out again the next thing are called wrist rotation so I'm going to have my arms by my side my hands are down and I'm going to make a light fist okay now I'm going to rotate those fists in towards my body

and then I'm going to rotate them out and away from the body and we're going to do that again in towards the body feel a stretch and away from the body we're going to do that one more time in towards the body and Away excellent okay now bring your arms out front you've still got that light wrist and then we're just going to rotate and up and the other way so it's just a little rotation for those wrists a little different way right you got it other way last time and release that okay so now we're going

to put our palms together okay we're going to open the book so you're hinging at the pinkies okay so I'm opening my book now the backs of the hands are going to go together and my fingertips are pointing towards me do you see what I'm doing there now the fingertips are going to go down towards the mat and then they're going to come out and away from me and they were going to bring them down again and towards up to the ceiling and close the book now we're going to use the thumb as the hinge okay so we're

opening backs of the hands together fingertips away fingertips down fingertips towards you fingertips to the ceiling and reverse it towards you down out up hinging at the thumbs bring the hands back together and release and stretch it out or Shake It Out let's just do a real quick little stretch for that wrist so all I'm doing is I'm just pulling gently on the palm there should feel pretty good let's release that and let's do the other side so the very last thing we're going to do before shavasana is we're going to bring

our knee up and in towards our chest okay just a little ankle rotation so all I'm doing is I'm taking my foot and I'm just rotating should feel good now if this bothers your knee you're going to grab behind the thigh okay so you don't have to have the shin you can have the thigh and then let's reverse it okay now I'm just going to grab my knee and I'm just going to bring it across the midline of the body super gentle here super gentle then I'm going to grab the knee I'm

going to hold on to the chair and I'm just going to open it okay and bring It Center and put that leg down and we're going to do the other side okay so we're going to grab that Shin or thigh either is fine just give it a little tug notice how I lengthen through my spine right crown of the head to the ceiling nice long spine here and then let's go ahead and do those ankle rotations first and reverse it should feel good oh that was that was my ankle that cracked I don't know if you heard that okay let's go ahead and grab our leg and we're just going to kind of bring it across the body stretch here you feel that yeah yeah and then we're going to open hold that chair that's fine just a little openness for that leg one more breath bring that knee in and place that foot on the floor all right I hope that felt good I thought it was a nice little series a little stretching series okay we're going to move back in our chair and we're getting ready for shavasana pose hands are going to rest lightly on

the thighs flip those Palms up to the ceiling close your eyes take a deep breath in and a full complete cleansing breath out keep Pace with life today is one day and tomorrow is another you don't have to eat it all drink it all say it all do it all right now do what's enough and then let it be pace yourself and know you'll have more opportunities in the days to come live each day as it arrives not before it appears not after it's gone you cheat yourself out of life when you rush ahead of it or linger behind it

bill each day with exactly one day's worth of living then do the same with the next day and the next Savor the moments the sensations the efforts the times and experiences with others always remember that too much is not preferable to enough give each bit of experience the time attention and Zeal that it deserves and that you deserve keep Pace with life and you'll enjoy all its Treasures to the highest degree take a deep breath in into full breath out drop your right ear towards your right shoulder

reach up with the right hand give the head a gentle tug pressing that left hand down towards the floor release it drop your chin towards your chest reach up with the hands give the head a gentle tug and release it drop your left ear towards your left shoulder reach up with the left hand give the head a gentle tug pressing that right hand down towards the floor release it look up just slightly open your mouth if you want to stretch your jaw bring your hands to your heart honoring one another we say namaste very well done we've already made it to

the end of day seven can you believe it do you agree with me that the hardest part is just getting to your chair and once we're here isn't it wonderful don't we feel great

DAY 8

let's get started so we're going to start by sitting up nice and tall and moving forward in our seat okay so we're not leaning back Focus just a moment on that mind and body and breath so let's ground our feet we've done this one now for a while so we kind of got the idea and let's ground those sits and Bones making sure they're connected to the Earth and equally weighted let's lift our heart lower our shoulders out of the ears place your hands lightly on the thighs flip the Palms up now close your eyes if that feels okay or you can just soften the Gaze if you'd rather connect to your heart center and just breathe

so taking just a moment here to connect to that breath feeling your natural inhalation and exhalation drawing your attention inward towards that Heart Center letting go of everything outside of the room we have one more breath here bring your hands to your heart set your intentions for today's practice one more breath here bring your hands back down to your thighs and open your eyes so how are you feeling just a little sense of calm and relaxation right doesn't that real good we're going to move into a next stretch

so we're going to drop our right ear towards our right shoulder just your natural range of motion here feeling that stretch and then we're going to tuck our chin so let that head fall chin towards the chest then we're going to go to the other side hi just a moment here feeling the stretch in the neck and let's do chanted chest one more time now we're going to look to the front of the room we're going to look to the right and we're going to look Center and we're going to look to the left

let's go ahead and look Center again and we're going to roll our shoulders so I want you to think about this shoulder roll as a very mindful movement right so we're really thinking about what's happening we're not just sitting here rolling the shoulders I want you to consciously connect right we talk about that bring let's go ahead and reverse it we talk about that mind body and breath connection so we can add that breathe in inhale as you come forward exhale as you come up and around

and I'll do that one more time so adding that breath in doing this mindfully and and release all right very very good we're going to come into a mountain pose so we'll bring our arms down by our side we've done this one before I know it's just such a good one to start with right we want to lengthen up through that spine but let's start here now we're going to come to goal post arms and we're going to squeeze those shoulder blades back behind us belly stays tight now let's

take our fingertips to the ceiling nice long think about lengthening through that spine right let's bring one hand down lengthen oh yeah and let's come down and let's do the other side lengthen and release maybe roll those shoulders again if you want to right that feel good nice long spine hear me thinking about long spine okay so now we're going to move into our cat and cow poses again this is a continuing to warm up that spine a little bit so for our cow pose today let's go ahead and grab the back of the

chair and then lengthen through the so I'm lifting up through my heart crown of the head to the ceiling and I'm squeezing my shoulder blades behind so my abdominals are tight here feel that stretch now let's move into our cat pose so we're going to round around letting the head fall tuck the chin let the head fall and then round through those shoulders right so A beautiful cat pose nice round spine let's come back up into cow pose again grab the back of that chair lifting up through the heart squeezing the shoulder

blades behind thinking about long spine and then round that cat yeah okay now we're gonna add the breath here we go inhale into your cow pose and exhale into your cat's pose again inhale into your cow pose and exhale into your cat pose one more time inhale into cow and move into that catapult all right let's come back up into seated position we should be feeling a nice little warmth happening in the center of the body as we continue to build a little bit of heat as we warm up so now we're going to do a little bit for the

lower part of the body so we'll do that seated Crescent lunge and we've done this one before we're going to take that right knee and we're going to open it so remember we stay just a moment here for a little stretch for the inner thigh now we're going to let that right excuse me that left knee fall down towards the mat letting that knee fall straight down okay so here we are in our beautiful Crescent lunge now if you would like just a little more Super gentle here we're warming up I'm going to push my foot

back so I'm up on those back toes and we'll push that foot back just a little bit okay so now I'm getting a little more stretch in the front side of that leg make sure you keep your heart lifted so the minute we begin to let that heart fall forward we're totally disengaging the stretch here okay so I would rather you have the heart lifted and the knee bent down you're going to just feel a little deep more stretch there okay one more breath here all right let's go ahead and face forward

we're going to do the other side now okay so we're going to take that left knee and open it up feel that stretch first right now we're going to let that knee fall down towards the floor so remember this is great position right here if this feels good for you heart is lifted knee straight down to the floor fine if you want a little bit more or if you feel like you know I don't know I don't really feel much of a stretch there then you're going to push that foot back just a little bit now you feel it a little more right

lifting that heart up feeling that stretch so trying to relax through this glute back here we tend to want to squeeze it and the more you relax it the more you're going to feel the stretch as well okay we just have one more breath and release that and let's face forward so we're going to move into a seated goddess pose all right so we're going to do a heel toe heel toe now in our goddess pose in our leg position we want the hips and the knees and the ankles and the toes to be in alignment okay so if you're feeling

like those knees are really wanting to fold in like it's just really hard for you to keep those open what I'd rather you do is heel toe the feet in a couple of times so that you can keep the alignment right I would rather that than have the feet wide and the knees fold in okay does that make sense all right let's get our feet positioned where we feel good now we're going to add our arms so let's go ahead and bring those arms up to goddess arms I call it gold post arms I don't know doesn't matter

right there it's the same movement right the same position for those arms so I want you to be squeezing your shoulder blades back behind you all right now we're gonna do a little at belly tight we're going to lean our goddess now are you feeling that sideways stretching right so we're working the side waist muscles and we're feeling a stretch and then we're going to come up Center and then we're going to lean the other way I know right feeling pretty good and let's come up let's do that one more

time lean come up lean the other way and come up now just bring your arms down take just a little break with the arms if you can leave the legs where they are let's do so continuing to get a little stretch if you really need to take a break I get it go ahead and bring your feet in it's okay all right let's go ahead and get those legs back in position if you've taken a little break with those legs let's come back up into those goddess arms okay now I'm going to twist right at the ribs keep these hips forward we're going

to twist to the right I know this knee wants to come forward doesn't it make sure this knee stays back and this hip stays down on that chair it wants to come forward don't let it we're going to come Center and twist the other way and come Center and lean and center and lean and Center Let's Twist to the left and center and twist to the right and Center last time lean and up and lean and up and release ah bring those feet ah how's that feel good all right we're going to come to standing behind our chair okay so go

ahead come up into a standing position and make your way back behind your chair so this is going to be our standing goddess pose we just did it seated and now we're going to do it standing so we'll take a heel toe heel toe okay so at least I want your legs to be the width of the chair legs preferably a little further if that feels okay for you your hands are just going to rest right here on the chair now just so you can see me a little bit better I'm going to go ahead and move out from behind my chair but I want you

to stay behind the chair so you've got that that chair for support okay so I'm going to come on on out and so here I am I'm going to do my heel toe and my heel toe all right so here's here's the width that I'm choosing for today now as we begin to move into our goddess legs what I want you to think about is pulling your belly in and tucking the pelvis okay so I'm just softening through that tailbone I'm lengthening that tailbone down and I'm pulling those abdominals in now I'm going to begin to soften the

knees right and I'm going to get let the hips the tailbone is down my front body lifts as I begin to bend those knees you feeling that so think about also another good cue is to roll to the outer edge of your feet so I'm I'm kind of rolling out with my feet my belly stays tight I'm lengthening down now here's a really important part is we want the hips the knees and the toes to be in alignment so remember seated we have the exact same thing we don't want those knees to fold in lifting up through that

pelvic floor can you deepen that squat oh yeah hello are you holding that chair right there's our goddess legs we have one more breath let's go ahead and straighten those legs and take just a moment how did that feel okay so we're going to move back into those goddess legs again and then we're going to let go of the chair and we're going to come into goddess arms now remember that's an add-on if you don't ever have to add on if you don't want to so if you want to keep your hands on the chair for

support it's fine if you want to come with me into God's arms fine okay are we ready heel toe heel toe so remember all of those things lift through the pelvic floor begin to lower lengthening through that tailbone belly is tight squeeze those pelvic floor muscles right okay are we ready we're gonna let go of that chair and we're going to come to those goddess arms belly is tight can you take that goddess legs any deeper and deeper into that squat right I'm rolling my feet out to the outer

edges of those feet my hips and knees and legs are in alignment my heart is lifted we have one more breath here let's go ahead and take a little break we've got another add-on here remember when we were seated we did our lean and our twist so we're going to add that on again hold that chair if that feels better for you okay are we ready let's do it this is it this is the last thing all right we're going to heel toe heel toe all right get those feet like you want them you're holding that chair now we're

going to begin to lower those hips back remember Bend at the knees pulling the belly in lifting through the heart lengthening through the tailbone rolling to the outer edge of those feet right got his arms here we go deep in that squat if you can let's do it we're going to lean and then we're going to come up and we're going to lean the other way I know I feel it too and they're going to come up let's twist and come Center and we're going to twist the other way and come Center straighten those legs

and come back ah how does that feel right okay so now we're going to do a horse pose so it's similar to goddess I'm sorry so we're going to do that same idea with our legs and then it's a little balance challenge okay so you're going to have that chair right there for support if you need it but we're going to be lifting the heel up off the floor and then we'll lift both heels off the floor okay just to kind of give you a sense of where we're headed it's called horse pose all right are we ready so let's

start with our heel toe heel toe we got this part down don't we right make sure those toes are pointed out of the diagonal begin to pull the belly in lengthen through the tailbone hips are down tailbone is long heart is lifted ribs are in are we ready for those goddess arms okay now remember hold on to that chair if you wish maybe to hold on to begin with and see how it feels but if you're feeling okay with me we're going to lift our right heel up off the mat and we're going to put it down we're

going to lift our left heel up off the mat and we're gonna put it down let's lift the left heel up and down right heel up and down right heel up and down left heel up and down listen here we go left heel up right heel up there's your balance belly tight down and down lift up and up whole breathe down and down up up hold breathe I know belly tight down down last one up up hold breath hold hold hold down down straighten those legs and come back into a seated position I know right pretty challenging goddess

and horse poses okay so let's give those legs a little stretch how do you how do you think let's take our right leg and lengthen it nice and long pyramid pose lengthen through the spine and let that heart fall forward ah that should feel pretty good and Tuck those chin and roll it up and let's do that again nice long spine come forward so remember look out don't look down right I'm looking out beyond my toes I'm keeping my back flat tuck that chin and roll it up we're gonna do that one more

time nice long spine forward we go and Tuck the chin and roll it up and let's go to the other side here we go stand nice and long through the spine let that heart fall forward keep the back flat don't round right this isn't cat this is Pyramid I'm looking out beyond my toes and roll it up and let's do that again nice long spine inhale to prepare exhale down we go and up we go inhale exhale and up we go very very good we're going to move back in our chair into shavasana pose hands are going to rest lightly on the

thighs flipping those Palms up close your eyes take a deep breath in and a full breath out take a deep breath in and a full complete cleansing breath Against the Wind when conditions are ideal you can make much progress yet even when conditions are not so favorable there are good and useful things you can do it's always great to have the encouragement support and assistance of others but even when you have little or no help you can move forward

you're wise to make the best of a good situation yet what's even more powerful is to make the best of a difficult situation sometimes the Winds of fate and circumstances are blowing your way great much of the time though you'll need to make your way Against the Wind sure you can claim the powerful headwind as an excuse and wait for better conditions and no one will blame you for that or you can go forward any way in the direction you've chosen and make progress in spite of the difficulties the situations events and people in this

world will not always align to push you ahead fortunately that never has to stop you take a deep breath in in a full breath out drop your right ear towards your right shoulder reach up with the right hand give the head a gentle tug as you press that left hand down towards the floor release it drop your chin towards your chest reach up with the hands giving the head a gentle tug release it drop your left ear towards your left shoulder

reach up with the left hand give the head a gentle tug pressing that right hand down towards the floor release it look up just slightly open your mouth if you want to stretch your jaw bring your hands to your heart

Please wait, Your Review is Very Important…

Dear Reader,

I hope this message finds you well. Thank you for choosing to read the 28 Day Chair Yoga for Seniors to Lose Weight. Your feedback is incredibly valuable to me, and I would love to hear your thoughts on the book. Whether you've just started, are halfway through, or have finished reading, your perspective matters.

Your feedback is immensely appreciated and will help me enhance future works.

Thank you for taking the time to share your thoughts on 28 Day Chair Yoga for Seniors to Lose Weight. Your support means the world to me.

Happy reading!

Carol Bolden

DAY 9

I'm so glad you've joined us today so you've made it it's day 9 of our 28 day chair yoga Journey we're going to start seated we'll move into a standing position for Mountain pose and triangle pose then we'll move back to seated now we're going to be using the block today and remember if you don't have a block you can substitute a big book and if you don't have that either it's fine just do the practice without it

okay now one thing you can do if you like is you can place that block back behind you on the seat so we're going to go ahead and move a little bit forward but if you want to you can lean back on that block and it still lets you sit up nice and tall and and so that's just an option if you don't want to do that that's fine too foreign just a little out sit up nice and Tall right so let's go ahead and take a moment to connect we're going to connect that mind and that body and that breath

right so getting our feet connected to the Earth grounding those feet thinking about grounding those sits bones so we already start with that connection right let's lift that heart lower the shoulders out of the ears placing the hands lightly on the thighs flip the Palms up close your eyes and then just connect to your heart center letting go of everything outside of the room just feeling your natural inhalation and exhalation begin to elongate the breath inhaling no more deeply exhaling a little more completely

and do that again just a couple more times and breathe normally bring your hands to your heart set your intentions for today's practice just one more breath here bring your hands back down to your thighs and open your eyes so we're going to bring our arms down by our side and then we're just going to lift our shoulders up into our ears and then we're going to drop let's do that again lift those shoulders up into the ears and let them drop one more time lift those shoulders up and let them drop

that should feel really good okay so we're gonna drop our right ear towards our right shoulder now I want you to reach up with the right hand and you're just going to lay the hand on the head you're not going to pull or tug it's just re you know kind of laying it there for a little weight now the opposite arm is going to extend out flexing through the wrist pushing through the palm oh yeah one more breath let's bring the hand down first then take the hand off of the head and then lift that head up

ah how does that feel let's go to the other side so we're going to let that left ear fall towards that left shoulder first just hang on here for a couple of breaths feeling that natural range of motion here and then we're going to lift that hand up and just lay it lightly on that head we're not pulling we're not tugging we're just letting the weight give us a little extra opposite arm is going to extend flexing through the wrist pushing through the palm one more breath here let's bring that hand down take the hand

off of the head and lift that head up oh my goodness how does that feel just a little movement in that neck right whatever natural movement you want to do I should feel pretty good okay coming into Mountain pose bring those arms down by your side spread those fingers nice and wide to stretch those hands come up into that GoPro storm squeezing those shoulder blades back behind you hands lengthening up towards the ceiling pulling the shoulders down trying to touch the ceiling with those fingertips one more breath bring the hands down

we're gonna do that one more time Mountain pose down we go spread goal post arm squeeze lengthen those arms to the ceiling make sure the shoulders are down out of the ears trying to touch the ceiling with those fingertips three two and one and release really really good okay so moving into our cat and our cow pose we're going to reach back and grab the back of that chair lifting up so I want you to think about lifting that through the throat right so nice open throat openness in the chest we're grabbing the back of that chair we're

squeezing out shoulder blades back behind us inhale to prepare exhale come down into your cat's pose hands on the thighs tuck the chin let the head fall now if you have your block behind you you can push your back into that block now we're going to lift up into cow pose again inhale in here and exhale into cat pose push that back into that block tucking that chin letting that head fall inhale into cow and exhale into count we're gonna do that one more time inhale into cow and exhale it again and release very good okay so we're

going to move a little bit further forward in our chair so you can leave that block right where it is you can set it on the floor if you prefer it's fine all right so we're going to do a heel and a toe and a heel and a toe now your hands are going to be on those thighs okay so let's check in with that alignment hip knee ankle toe right so we want everything in alignment knees are not folding in knees are wide hands are on the thighs where we're going to begin to let our heart fall forward okay so holding onto those

thighs giving yourself a little support pull your belly in nice and tight now we're going to drop our right shoulder between our legs you feel the stretch there on that upper shoulder and back upper arm right I even get a little bit into the upper back feels pretty good and up we go and then we're gonna do the other side and then up we go okay so let's take just a moment now we're going to do that again and let's have the breath see how if we can connect that breath in with that movement all right nice conscious

remember keep the Mind involved we want to keep everything that that mindfulness if you will nice long spine hands on those thighs inhale exhale we're gonna let that heart fall forward inhale exhale let that left shoulder fall inhale up exhale other shoulder Falls inhale up exhale shoulder Falls one more and remember if using the yoga breath makes you dizzy leave it out just breathe naturally it's okay right so we don't ever want to do anything to create any discomfort and up we go all right all the way up so if that goes true

anytime we're using the breath right if that just really doesn't work for you or you're beginning to feel light-headed or whatever just read normally leave it out it's okay just don't hold your breath okay so now let's go ahead and bring those feet in just taking a little break here I should have done that while I was talking sorry okay so the next pose is called malasana with Garland pose so we're going to take those feet back wide again all right so let's do this again so a heel toe and a

heel toe now it's probably not quite as wide as we did just a minute ago so don't feel like you've got to get those feet just as wide as you can and you'll see why here in just a second all right we've got our hands on those thighs we're going to let that heart fall forward again so keeping the back flat right so we're looking out not down now I'm going to put the fleshy part of my arm right in here on the fleshy part of that inner thigh and then the other side and then I'm going to bring my

Palms together so the idea here is a yin yang kind of thing right I'm going to push in with my legs and I'm going to push out with my arms alright so feeling that pressure pressing in with my legs pressing out with my arms we have one more breath here let's release that come up and just take those legs in for a moment does that feel okay can we do that again let's do it okay we're going to do a heel toe out we're going to hinge forward bring our elbows to the inside of those knees Palms are facing together

squeeze the inner thighs in pressing the arms away activating inner and outer thighs is what you should be feeling one more breath here and release all right very good let's go ahead and bring those feet in okay so now we're going to move into seated triangle and we're actually going to use our block now for on you you're like we haven't used our block yes we're going to use our block in this one but we're not going to use it to begin with we're going to start without it and then

we're going to add it in so with your right leg we're going to do a heel toe and a heel toe okay so now we've got that alignment right we kind of got that down you know we need to make sure that that's in alignment this leg stays right where it is we're going to bring our arms up kind of those Warrior two arms we haven't really talked about that yet we will okay so my arms are parallel to the floor alright so often what I'll see in my in-person classes is maybe this or maybe that so just take a moment to

really get those arms in alignment with the parallel to the floor and then I want you to think about pulling your shoulders down so often we end up here right so we're going to pull those shoulders down our belly is tight now moving only at the rib cage the upper body is going to move towards this knee that we've extended out so here's our version of triangle pose right here and then we're going to bring those ribs in center and let's do that again so we're really trying to disconnect the upper body and the lower

body so the lower body is staying stable it's not moving and then the upper body is moving let's do that one more time you feeling it can you feel the how the upper body only is moving and Center let's bring those arms down let's bring that foot in so now we're going to do the other side okay so we're going to take this left leg and we'll do a heel toe and a heel toe so again check on that alignment this leg stays right where it is bring those arms out so think about squeezing your muscles

against the bones in the arm so if I came up to you and I tried to pull your arm down I wouldn't be able to so I want you to activate those arms right so it's very active pose even though we're static we're just hanging out here it's still a very active pose right okay are we ready just the ribs out we go and Center let's do that again rib cage only remember upper body is separate from the lower body and Center we have one more just like that and Center we go bring the arms down and bring that foot in okay so checking in how did that feel so that's a great version and that you want to stick with that version you're going to stick with that version now if you're with me I'm gonna go right now I'm going to grab my block and I'm going to set it here so you'll see here in a moment let's go ahead and heel tie this foot out okay now my block is right here by my foot okay we're going to bring those arms up now we're going to remove that upper body is moving and then I'm going to bring that hand down to the block okay so what do I do if I don't have a block you're going to hold either you can have your hand on your leg or you can just have it down by the side okay so if you want to have it on the block that's great if you don't have that block it can be down or it can be on your leg okay all right are we ready we're going to come back up and then we're going to bring those ribs Center and we're going to bring the arms down Okay so we're gonna do that one more time just like that ready here we go up

ribs hand comes down beautiful triangle pose now here's the thing about triangle pose often you'll kind of want to let your heart sink forward see how I'm kind of letting that shoulder fall down so I don't want you to do that I want you to lift up so now I'm making my side waist muscles work here right I'm lifting up so I've got an alignment of wrist shoulder shoulder and wrist how's that feel one more breath here let's come up notice how my ribs are still to the side let's come Center

and down down okay bringing that foot in we're gonna do the other side now so this hand is going to be uh or I'm sorry the block is going to be out here so let's do a heel toe and a heel toe okay so get that all set bring those arms up okay are we squeezing we have those upper arms are we squeezing these away things squeezing okay are we ready now let's just bring the ribs out now you're gonna just kind of tilt forward maybe the hand comes to the block lifting up through the chest maybe you

look up if that feels okay on your neck if you don't have to block your hand is on the leg or it's just hanging out on the side one more breath bring come up bring those ribs in bring the hands back to the heart back to the heart back to the legs to your lap and we're gonna do that again let's do it bring it up squeeze we got this ribs only and down we go lifting up now one thing you can do if you want is you can put this hand right here on the waist and lift Your Heart Right making sure that heart stays lifted and then

you can add that arm let's come back up and in we go and hands come down all right very very good now just set your block aside if you have it we're going to come back to it in just a moment but now we're going to come to standing all right on the right side of our chair so it's all come up to standing and we're going to come here to the right side of the chair I'm just going to go ahead and set my block in my in the seat of my chair kind of get it out of my way all right so we're going to start with our feet

hit distance apart so this means that as you look down you're you're in alignment right your hips are right in alignment with those legs we're going to come into that mountain pose so bring those arms down by your side spreading the fingers nice and wide come back to those goal post arms squeeze your shoulder blades all right now we're going to extend our Mountain pose fingertips to the ceiling with your right hand I want you to grab your left wrist and lean lengthen up towards the ceiling and then we're going

to lean our Mountain and then we're going to come up and we're going to grab the opposite wrist lengthen and lean our Mountain and up we go now let's release and we're going to do that again and we're going to add a Twist okay so Mountain pose spread your fingers go post arms squeeze those shoulder blades back behind you belly is tight lengthen up right hand is going to grab left wrist lengthen let's learn our mountain now I want you to turn and look up at the ceiling take the twist out come up grab the

opposite wrist lengthen first up to the ceiling lean and then we're going to twist and look up take the twist out come back up and release that okay how's that feel pretty good I'm just rolling my shoulders a little bit because that feels good so we're going to move into a standing triangle pose we will be using the block again if you don't have the block you're just going to use your leg so we're going to turn I'm going to face the seat of our chair now we're going to take this leg that's

next to the chair and you're going to step it under just just slightly under the chair opposite leg is going to step back hips come forward so my hips are around facing the seat of the chair okay see how that feels alright really really good now holding on to that chair we're going to turn so that our hips are facing forward front knees straight does that make sense kind of so the back foot is is back at that 45 degree angle the front leg is straight and we're going to bring those arms up nice okay we're gonna hinge over

and then we're going to bring our hand down maybe you've got the the Block in the seat of the chair that's a great option right the hand is there on the seat of the chair there's a beautiful triangle pose now if you'll notice my wrist shoulder shoulder wrist are in alignment here if you don't have the the block your hand's going to be in the seat of the chair okay all right we're going to come up and then we're gonna bring those ribs centered and we're going to bring the

hands down okay we're going to do that one more time all right here we go up we go squeeze the muscles against the bones and the arms activating that upper body upper body moves over that chair the hand drops down to the seat of the chair or the Block open nice and open feeling that inner thigh stretching one more breath come back up Center and release okay let's take a little break here so we'll go to the other side so we have one more thing to add to that triangle pose but let's go ahead and start here

and do the other side so I've moved to the other side of my chair remember I'm going to start I just kind of want to get those hips around kind of feeling that front leg straight then I'm going to move those hips out to face me bring the arms up okay so front leg is straight now as my ribs come forward do you notice how this hip is kind of hiking up a little bit then I'm going to bring my hands down if I've got my block they're going to be on that block I'm lifting up so this is a pretty decent stretch on

that inner thigh you feel it okay keep the front leg straight I know you want to bend it keep it straight come back Center and then those ribs come Center let's do that one more time ribs come over the chair drop the hand down lifting up one more breath here we're going to press up bring the rib Center and down we go all right how did that feel there is more to that triangle pose but for today we're going to leave it at that and then maybe another day we'll add a couple more things to that try to that triangle

pose but I want to start there all right very very good so now the next thing we're going to do and I'm going to just kind of set my block aside for now get it out of my way so now the next thing we're going to do is a downward facing dog we're going to start with our downward facing puppy so what I want to make sure is that your chair is on carpet or it's on a sticky mat like a yellow mat something that's going to keep that chair from sliding okay so we don't want the chair moving and so the other thing

to think about is I want you to think about pressing down not out okay so the first thing we'll do is with our I'm going to turn my chair to the side you stay facing me you're behind your chair okay so what I'm going to do is I'm going to take a step back from my chair my hands are on the chair see how long my arms are right and then I'm going to hinge I'm hinging at the hips so I'm not bending my at the waist right I'm hinging at the hips my arms are on that chair now as I'm coming into my down dog I'm

going to take one more step back and I'm going to begin to let my heart fall forward okay so my heart is falling between my my arms and I'm just letting my upper body sink I'm shooting my hips back behind me my head is forward and I have one more breath here and let's go ahead and roll it up into a standing position okay so that that is version one of your down dog and it's a great version okay so let's do that one more time let's go ahead and step back so what I like to do is begin to let my

heart fall forward see how my elbows now are bending so I'm going to go ahead and take one more little step back so that my arms are nice and straight let that heart fall forward make sure my hips are back I have one more breath here belly is super tight as I come up to a standing position take a step forward okay so that's a great version and I would encourage you that that feels good for you stick with it if you want to come with me we're going to move into using the side of our chair so let's go

ahead and move to the side of our chair now so you'll see the difference pretty quickly all right so you'll see if you feel like sticking with this one if you want to go back to your hands behind the chair so let's take a little step back okay now we're going to hinge again you're hinging at the hips not the waist hinge at the hips we're going to bring our hands to the seat of the chair and bring your weight forward okay now we're going to start in puppy and the reason we do that is it just it's

going to give us a good stretch in the back but it takes out those the stress on the wrists okay so let's go ahead and bring our forearms down onto the chair okay now the idea here is you want your hips to go up high and your heart to go back towards your thighs okay so see what's happening here I'm pressing my heart back and my hips up so I have one more breath here let's go ahead and come up step forward take a little break roll up into a standing position so how did that feel okay so checking in I know it's a pretty good

stretch for the hamstrings that's what it's for Rise the back side no the whole back side of the body it's not just hamstrings but I feel it a lot in my hamstring so one thing you can do if it's really like okay this is just too much for me he's bend the knees a little and that's okay right all right so let's try that again just like that and then we're going to add one final thing on all right so I'm taking a little step back right I'm going to hinge here at my hips I'm going to place my hands in the chair

I'm going to bring my weight forward now I'm going to lower onto my forearms but I want to keep my shoulders right over those elbows okay so I'm not so I've got this alignment happening now I'm going to take a little step back and as I begin to press my heart back my hips High and if you want to bend the knees a little bend the knees a little feeling the stretch in the back side of the body I feel a stretch in the arms the shoulders this is such a nice one downward facing puppy one more breath here and then let's come

up okay step forward step forward roll up nice and slow okay now here's the thing if having your head down is making you dizzy what I want you to do is not let the head fall as far so the head will end up staying above the heart okay and that's fine too now the final piece of this is instead of being on our forearms for downward facing puppy we're going to be on our hands for downward facing dog and you'll feel the difference so only if it works for you so let's go ahead and take one step back to start with we're going to

place our hands in the seat of the chair and bring our weight forward now I'm going to take another pretty good size step back now do you feel where the chair could be sliding right it won't for long so now we're going to press the hips up shoot the hips up high heart back feeling that stretch now if you want to take another little step back I'm going to take another step back and I'm going to get my heart even lower there we go so for me this feels good this is a good downward facing dog for

me I want you to do what works for your body feeling that stretch in the back side of the legs the back side of the body hips are high heart is back we've got three and two and one now listen as you come up take a step forward hold that chair roll it up nice and slow how did that feel okay let's come to seated okay excellent excellent excellent just take a little break a little breath here right ah so we're gonna move into Crescent lunge we're going to take that right knee and we're going to open it nice and wide and

we're going to let our left knee fall down towards the floor pushing the foot back behind you a little bit relaxing this glute feeling the stretch in the front side of that leg let's release that and we'll do that again back of the kneecap towards the ceiling facing forward and face forward while I sit facing forward I met forward that way now we're going to face forward this way towards me I need to be a little clearer with my cues don't I all right let's lengthen through the spine on an inhale exhale we're going to let

that heart fall forward pyramid pose keep the back flat looking beyond the toes tuck the chin and roll it up and let's do that again nice long spine let that heart fall forward oh that feels so good and up we go let's do the other side here we go open it up nice and wide let that knee fall down towards I don't know why I'm singing let that knee fall down towards the mat looking over this front leg I'll cue that a little bit better belly tight let's release and let's do that one more

time so kind of pushing the back of the kneecap towards the ceiling a little bit there feeling that stretch right one more breath and release we got to do our pyramid pose so let's extend that leg out lengthen through the spine let the heart fall forward keep the back flat look beyond your toes and let's come up we'll add that breath inhale to extend exhale to hinge forward one more time inhale up exhale forward and up weaker very good let's go ahead and move into strip Austin a pose so leaning back

hands resting lightly on the thighs flip the Palms up to the ceiling take a deep breath in and a full breath out let's inhale here and as you exhale go ahead and close your eyes live at your highest level right now allow strength to Surge within you notice the power of confidence as it rises from deep inside and bursts through all your awareness feel enthusiasm Gathering within and aiming you toward your best possibilities be energized by the courage that steadily streams out from your most profound purpose

ride upon the newness of this moment as the Miracle of Life pervades your whole existence invigorate your most honest thoughts and transform them into valuable action all the while project a sincere and peaceful presence in what you do engage in life with an endless reservoir of kindness and understanding Embrace every opportunity for joy Marvel at the beauty and wonder that surrounds you all the time let it all unfold naturally generously without worry or desperation give life your best and live at your highest level

take a deep breath in and a full breath out drop your right ear towards your right shoulder reach up with the right hand give the head a gentle tug pressing that left hand down towards the floor release it drop your chin towards your chest reach up with your hands give the head a gentle tug release it drop your left ear towards your left shoulder reach up with the left hand give the head a gentle tug pressing that opposite hand down towards the floor release it look up just slightly open your mouth if you want to stretch your jaw bring your hands to your heart.

DAY 10

let's get started okay so we're going to start with that same connection of mind and body and breath right so we're moving forward in our chair we're not leaning back Place both feet on that floor and feel the sits bones grounded to the chair right let's place our hands lightly on our thighs flip the Palms up to the ceiling close your eyes and connect to the breath feeling your natural inhalation and exhalation and then we're going to move that breath down into our diaphragm as we inhale the belly extends we're filling the lungs from the bottom up

and as we exhale we actively pull the belly button in towards the spine pushing the air up and out of the lungs do that again inhale and exhale one more time inhale breathe normally bring your hands to your heart set your intentions for today's practice one more breath here bring your hands down to your thighs and open your eyes and we're going to roll our shoulders so it's a mindful movement right feeling that sensation of that forward and up and back and down and then let's reverse it nice one more

all right so we're going to go ahead and grab the back of our chair all right so link think about lifting up through the chest shoulders are down and back behind you now we're going to drop our right ear towards our right shoulder just a little different way of stretching into the neck you feel it dropped it chin towards the chest and then we're going to do left ear to left shoulder and then we're going to do chanted chest now release the chair bring your hands to the back of your head and just let

the elbows hang towards the floor a little weight here not pulling no tugging on that head just letting the weight of the hands and the shoulders and the elbows give you a little more stretch one more breath bring the hands down to the thighs and lift the head up and let's roll those shoulders again how does that feel excellent work okay moving into Mountain pose bring those arms down by the side spread those fingers nice and wide let's come into those goal post arms squeezing those shoulder blades back

behind now we're going to lengthen our fingertips towards the ceiling now we're going to do a little add-on here so I'm going to bring my right hand to the chair I'm going to lengthen nice and long and then I'm going to lean my mountain take your hand and I want you to lift it up towards the ceiling turn and look up and then we're going to lean that mountain again and then we're going to take our hand and we're going to look up at the ceiling one more time lean hand up to the ceiling bring the hand

down and we're going to do that whole thing again here we go Mountain pose go post arms fingertips to the ceiling left hand down right hand extends try to touch the ceiling with those fingertips hold that chair and let's lean that mountain feel a stretch in the side waist take the hand up to the ceiling turn and look up and lean hand to the ceiling turn and look up one more lean hand to the ceiling turn and look up and release very very good okay so let's bring our hands to our heart and I want you to think about lifting up through

the spine and opening up through that throat now we're going to move into cow pose from here bellies stays tight take your thumbs to the back wall see we were already prepped and ready for that cow pose Now Catch pose we're going to round pull the belly in pull those ribs back round through the spine tuck the chin let the hands fall to the lap and let's do that again thinking about lifting up opening through the throat thumbs to the back wall let's inhale into cowl exhaling to calf inhale into cow

and exhale into calf and release okay so that's a great version of cat and cow we're going to do a little different version now we're going to take our hands and we're going to place them behind our head elbows are wide so again we're lifting nice and long through the spine we're open through the throat we're going to inhale here and then as we exhale into cat's pose we're going to let those elbows fall down towards the floor keep the hands behind the head a little bit of a stretch here let the

head fall inhale we're going to lift those elbows up towards uh up and we're going to open up through the chest and then exhale we're going to come down so we're just tucking that chin we're letting that those elbows give us the weight of the elbows give us a little deeper stretch into that neck let's do that one more time inhale up we go there's your inhale and exhale down we go can we do it one more time inhale up exhale down and release very very good so we're going to keep our knees facing forward

remember how we grounded those feet to begin with so we're going to keep those feet grounded to the Earth knees are forward hips are forward we're going to take our right hand and we're going to place it on the outside of that left knee let's take the other hand back to the seat of the chair we're going to lengthen through the spine we're going to pull out shoulder back and turn and look over that shoulder and face forward okay we're going to do the other side now so it's just a super gentle seated twist this hand is going to come to the outside of that knee opposite hand back by the chair lengthen pull the shoulder back turn and look and release I want to do that one more time so just paying attention making sure your knees are staying forward hand comes to the outer edge of the leg opposite hand to the chair lengthen pull the shoulder back turn and look over that left shoulder maybe you take the Gaze a little further so it's not necessarily the head just the eyes just take the Gaze a little further

and phase four we're gonna do that one more time on the other side so I'm not moving my head any further opposite hand back I'm just taking my eyes extend through the spine pull the shoulder back so we're turning and we're looking first so just do your natural stretch here then if you can take your gaze a little further over that right shoulder one more breath here and release okay very good so we're going to do a different version of a seated forward fold and then we're going to add a little movement in with that forward fold it's called revolving so we're going to go ahead and sit back in our chair so that the seat of the chair is between our legs okay feeling alright so just hang out here for a moment kind of get that feeling now both of my Palms are right in the seat of that chair okay that's what's going to give us the support we're going to pull our belly in we're going to lengthen through the spine and we're going to begin to let that heart fall forward so again my back is flat

I'm looking out not down and then I'm going to tuck my chin and I'm going to roll up let's do that again nice long spine inhale to prepare exhale begin to come forward tuck that chin and roll it out okay so now we're going to revolve our forward fold so we're going to take our right hand and we're just going to kind of move it in just a little bit so it's right under your eyesight okay now we're going to extend through the spine we're going to come forward now this left arm is going to twist open

so again this is not too too deep of a Twist okay so I don't want my arm to be way out here I want the action to happen at the ribs okay so the shoulders are in alignment so my wrist my shoulder and my shoulder are right in alignment I'm looking up at the hand towards the ceiling if that feels okay on your neck if that doesn't feel okay then you're just going to look out now we're going to bring that right excuse me that left hand down and then we're going to replace the other opposite hand and we're going to revolve the other way again making sure that wrist shoulder shoulder are in alignment right belly is tight one more breath let's bring that hand down and we're going to roll it up into a seated position okay so that's a great version and if you want to stick with that version you're going to stick with it if you want a little bit more we're going to instead of our hands being here in the chair it's going to be our forearms okay all right so let's nice and long through the spine inhale to prepare exhale we're

going to begin to let that heart fall forward and then we're going to bring those forearms to the chair okay how does that feel right letting your heart fall a little further if that feels okay now we're going to bring that left shoulder right all right that left elbow excuse me kind of right in the middle and then I'm going to open up so it's a little deeper twist right but I've still got my wrist shoulder and shoulder in alignment I'm not over extending that upper arm one more breath here bring

that elbow back to the mat to the chair and open the other way one more breath here go ahead and bring that elbow down can we do it one more time on each side let's do it we've got this are you feeling the stretch on the inner thighs right at the waist I'm feeling all kinds of things stretching down we go let's do the other side and down we go place your hands on the seat of the chair and then roll up nice and slow how did that feel like bring those legs in why right quite a stretch I know I know okay we're gonna move into

a Warrior Two pose then we're going to reverse our Warrior and we're going to move into a side angle pose all right so we're going to take our right knee and we're going to do our heel now you know what we're going to take our right knee and we're going to do a full open that's what I want to do for this one so you see what I did there I just grabbed that knee and I opened it all the way so it's at that 90 degrees right so we've got one knee is facing me and one knee is at 90 degrees facing the

wall beside me now you're going to turn so that you're about at the ribs the hips stay stable on the chair you're going to turn and you're going to bring those arms out so there is a beautiful Warrior Two pose okay so now we're going to reverse the warrior so this is the hand that's considered the front hand so the right we're going to flip that Palm up to the ceiling now you're going to take that hand and you're going to lift it up as high as you can towards the ceiling your

other hand is coming to the chair for support Lift Up Lift Up Lift up now come past the midline of the body there's that reverse Warrior let's come back to that Warrior Two squeeze the muscles against the bones in the arms squeeze

squeeze squeeze and let's release that and let's bring that leg in okay so how did that feel okay let's do the other side so we're going to go ahead and come to the other side bring those arms out so remember shoulders need to stay down out of the ears we're squeezing the

muscles against the bones and the arms we're activating that upper body let's look over those left fingertips flip that Palm up to the ceiling and then we're going to reverse our Warrior so remember we want to go up as high as we can as much to the ceiling as we can and then bring that hand past the midline of the body and there's our reverse Warrior we're going to come back to that Warrior Two and we're going to bring our hands down and face forward okay so we're going to do that same thing

again and we're going to add a side angle pose and then we're going to add an extended side angle pose so it'll be really feeling very good on the sideways it'll do good stretches so let's take that knee and we're going to open it we're going to bring those arms out to the side we've done this one right let's reverse our Warrior Flip that Palm up and back grab that chair now we're going to come back to our Warrior two and then we're going to let that right arm FL come down to the right

leg Palm faces up open up through the chest see what I did there I opened up so I'm not letting myself sink down I'm lifting up make my side waist muscles do that work now if you want just a little bit more the hand that's in the air you're going to bring it over so I call this bicep by ear you see kind of how that that happens all right inhale to prepare and exhale we're going to Windmill back to that Warrior Two we're going to reverse our Warrior up and back we're going to come back to that Warrior

Two and release Face Forward okay we gotta do the other side ready here we go open that leg up come into that Warrior Two let's flip that Palm up and back reverse our Warrior back to Warrior Two now we're going to go to side angle pose so I'm just flipping my palm up my arm is resting on that thigh my wrist shoulder and shoulder are in alignment for that side angle pose and then we can extend our side angle pose we have one more breath let's press back to that Warrior Two reverse it one more time

back to Warrior Two and release and face forward ah doing okay all right we're gonna come to standing on the right side of our chair okay and we're gonna face the seat of the chair here okay so we're going to the leg that's next to the back of the chair we're going to take that foot and we're going to place it right under the seat of the chair now when you bend this knee I want it to touch okay but I want you to be able to bend the knee opposite leg is going to take a step back and you're at that for that leg that

foot is at that 45 degree angle so it's not way out here you want the toes to come forward heel is down bring those ribs around bend your front knee bring your hands to Heart all right now we're going to extend our arms to the ceiling and then we're going to turn and face me into a Warrior Two there you go alright so this knee is tracking right at your second toe so the knee is open bring the ribs to the center of the body flip this Palm up towards the ceiling we're going to reverse that Warrior

all the way up looking up if that feels okay on your neck now we're going to come back to Warrior two and then we're going to put that left hand down in the chair this is our side angle pose so again lifting up through the heart belly is tight make your side waist muscles work here extend that side angle if you wish okay we're gonna have windmill starting with this hand here inhale to prepare exhale windmill all the way up do you feel that side waist working hard flip that Palm up and back back to that Warrior Two

grab the chair and release good work let's do the other side okay we're gonna do it so we're going to start facing the chair with that foot remember it's the foot with the next to the back of the chair otherwise you're going to be turning and it's going to be very uncomfortable and so the foot next to the back of the chair that's the one that goes under take a step back hips are forward bend the front knee okay let's take our hands out and then we're going to move into that Warrior

Two I don't know I move this foot just a little bit didn't I write that's okay so that knee is attracting to that second toe my hips are forward my belly is tight my ribs are in the center of the body so to tend to kind of want to go forward so we want to really consciously make sure that our head neck spine are all in alignment pull those shoulders down out of the ears squeeze the muscles against the bones and the arms look over those right fingertips flip the right palm to the ceiling and reverse your Warrior

remember ceiling first touching the ceiling then come past the midline of the body looking up if that feels okay on your neck back to that Warrior two then hand to the chair for side angle pose lifting up extend that side angle if you wish one more breath now we're going to Windmill back to that Warrior Two there's our power move let's reverse that Warrior One More Time feel that sideways stretching come back and release very good did that feel okay excellent okay we're going to stay on this side of the chair and we're going

to do so this is a heart opening with eagle arms okay so it's not Eagle pose but we're going to do a little heart opening here so we're going to take my hands and I'm going to interlace my fingers behind my back all right now I want you to push those Knuckles down and away okay so thinking about pressing down pulling those shoulder blades back opening up through the chest let's take a deep breath in and out now I'm going to bring my arms I'm going to open wide I want you to press back

squeeze those shoulder blades behind starting with your right arm you're going to cross on top of that right arms on top give yourself a hug lift the elbows to the ceiling on an inhale exhale we're going to let those elbows come down and we're going to begin to just kind of fall forward knees are bent Whispering those elbows Center and then we're going to open and then we're going to cross the opposite arm take the elbows to the ceiling take the elbow Center elbows back down now listen we're going to come up

and then we're going to bring our arms up into a v looking up come up until your tiptoes one more breath bring your hands down hands behind the back press those Knuckles back open up through that chest bring those arms out to the side left arm on top hug yourself um lift those elbows up towards the ceiling belly tight elbow Center elbows go down elbows Center open right arm on top hug yourself oh yeah it feels good up we go and Center down we go elbow center now we're going to release those arms up to the ceiling we're going

to come up onto those tippy toes looking up if that feels okay belly tight one more breath and down we got a little balance work there at the end didn't we yeah I pulled that one out on you now I didn't even give you a little heads up that we were doing that did we okay alright so this next pose is called I didn't say this but I actually came to my seat so I'm hoping that you followed me I didn't say to come to your chair did I all right so this next pose is called half lord of the fishes so

we're going to take our right knee we're going to open it nice and wide we're going to take our left arm and open it and then we're going to bring that arm all the way across grab the chair now this is important lengthen through the spine turn and look over the back of your chair one more breath let's do that again open keep this knee open don't let it fold in bring it across lift and twist one more breath here let's release that and face forward so now I'm going to take this this left leg I'm going to bring it up so I'm going to bring my ankle on top of my knee now I'm going to give you options so if this doesn't feel good for you this is Pigeon pose if this one doesn't this version of pigeon puzzle doesn't feel good so here's your options you've got two other options one option is you're going to leave this leg right where it is and you're going to cross ankle the ankle okay the other option is you're going to extend your right leg and you're going to place your ankle on the shin okay so you've got two options there I'm personally going to be here okay I'm going to lengthen nice and long through my spine and I'm going to begin to let my heart fall forward just super gentle here keep the back flat look out not down tuck that chin and roll it up let's move this knee up and down just a little bit so that is moving the hip joint let's do that again nice long spine heart comes forward look out not down pigeon pose you feeling your hip right back in here me too and round very good okay we gotta

do the other side so now we're going to take that left knee and open it half lord of the fishes bring that right arm out and across the body grab the chair lengthen through the spine turn and look over the back of your chair keeping that right knee open don't let it fold in open it up and let's do that again bring it across the body grab the chair lift and twist one more breath here and release okay face forward pigeon pose on this side so again you've got options this is option number one this is the one I'm going to do you've also got the option of ankle to ankle and you've got the option of ankle to shin okay so pick what version you like and let's just hang out here for a moment in our pigeon pose we're going to lengthen through the spine keeping the back flat begin to let that heart fall forward all right tuck the chin and roll it up and then just move that knee up and down a little bit and then let's do that one more time nice long spine belly tight let that heart fall forward and roll it up all right let's move into

shavasana pose so we're going to sit back in our chair you can lean back now if you wish place your hands lightly on the thighs flip the Palms up towards the ceiling close the eyes take a deep breath in and a full breath out the first step are you hesitant to take the first step because you're worried it could be the wrong one most likely that first step won't be in exactly the ideal Direction but that's no reason to worry because it's just the first step you will learn from it and then be able

to take a much more experienced and informed step you're not going to make a perfect start nonetheless you must make a start if you're going to get anything done so go ahead and get it over with whether it works well or whether it doesn't it gets you moving the more you act the more effective each additional action will become get the process started and get that upward spiral in motion make the first step as good as you can don't fret that it's not perfect let it get you started and you'll find

you can handle it very well from there take a deep breath in and a full breath out drop the right ear towards the right shoulder reach up with the right hand give the head a gentle tug pressing that left hand down towards the floor release it drop your chin towards your chest reach up with the hands give the head a gentle tug release it drop the left ear towards the left shoulder reach up with the left hand give the head a gentle tug pressing that opposite hand down towards the floor release it

look out just slightly open your mouth if you want to stretch your jaw bring your hands to your heart

DAY 11

let's get started so we're going to sit up nice and tall in our chair right moving forward we've done this one many times now it's just that moment that we have right to focus on that mind and that body and the breath so we're going to ground our feet to the Earth thinking about having both feet on the floor equally weighted and then the same thing with those sits bones right we have those grounded to the chair we're not leaning one way or the other we're gonna lift our heart out lower those shoulders out of the ears place the hands lightly on the thighs flip those Palms up to the ceiling we're going to close our eyes and then just begin to notice your natural breath right so just that natural inhalation and exhalation

we're going to move that breath down into the diaphragm so we move from that shoulder breath to that belly breath so we're going to inhale feeling the lungs from the bottom up that belly will extend and exhale pull the belly button in actively pushing the air up and out of the lungs so do that again inhale and exhale one more inhale and exhale let's breathe normally now we're going to continue with our diaphragmatic breath and we're going to inhale to four counts and exhale to five so it'll be something like this inhale two three four exhale two three four five inhale two three four exhale two three four five and breathe normally bring your hands to your heart set your intentions for today's practice bring your hands back down to your thighs and open your eyes let's look over that right shoulder and like Center and let's look over that left shoulder and Center we're going to do that one more time okay so as you look over the that right shoulder don't move the head

further I want you to just move the eyes just the Gaze a little bit further and face Center and let's do the other side so it's just a little gaze continuing with that gaze one more breath here and face forward excellent work we're going to bring our hands down by our side and do our shoulder shrugs so our shoulders are shrugging up into our ears and then we're going to just let them fall let gravity help there shrug them up and fall one more time shrug them up and just let her fall good work okay so

we're going to drop our right ear towards our right shoulder and I'm just going to lift my right hand and I'm going to place it lightly on my head and I'm just going to feel a little extra stretch there because of the weight of that hand one more breath let's bring our hand down bring the head up now I'm going to tuck my chin and I'm going to reach up with my hands just lightly they're going to just lay on the back of my head as my elbows are towards the floor and they're giving a little

bit so with the weight of the arms and a little bit of gravity you should feel a little more stretch into the back of that neck remove the hands first and then lift the head up and let's go to the other side so hang out here for just a moment right feeling the stretch and then we're going to reach up with the hand and we're just going to lay it lightly on that head ah just feeling the nice stretch into the shoulder I should the shoulder it's really the neck isn't it well that's where I feel

it anyway one more breath bring the hand off of the head first and then we're going to lift that head up now all I want you to do is just lift your head up so just a little bit of openness through the throat right just a nice little stretch there one more breath and face forward okay very good we're going to move into Mountain pose I know you're like okay we do mountain pose a lot but it's just a great one to to warm up it's just a really good one so yes we're doing Mountain pose again let's come down so

spread those fingers see how that feels right stretching out that hand those fingers coming into goal post arms now we release the finger stretch when we move into those gold post arms or goddess arms I'm squeezing my shoulder blades back behind fingertips to the ceiling nice long hands up shoulders are down one more breath let's release it we're going to do that again Mountain pose we've got this gopost arms squeeze those shoulder blades back behind you belly tight lengthening those hands to the ceiling

shoulders stay down think about can you lengthen any more through that spine right can you stretch any more one more breath and bring those arms down so that one looks like you're just hanging out with your hands in the air but it's a very active pose do you feel that right if you really work at lengthening through and just trying to lengthen that spine it's a very active pose we're going to move into our cow pose and Cat pose again I know we do them a lot but it's just a really good way to

warm up that spine so we're going to do it by grabbing the back of the chair and lifting up through the chest squeezing those shoulder blades back behind you so I'm going to look up just slightly I'm opening up through that throat my belly is tight abdominals engaged all right are we ready let's round down into that cat pose hands to the thighs tuck the chin looking down at my lap make sure you're letting your head fall so I'm not holding my head up right I'm letting that head fall really tucking

that chin let's do that again and we'll add the breath let's inhale into our cow pose grabbing the back of the chair if that feels okay and then exhale into your cat pose again inhale into cow and exhale into cap inhale into cow and exhaling to calf last time let's do it make it count really feel that stretch exhale down we go and release okay so we're gonna come into goal post arms right so we've done this one before we know we're pretty good uh idea of where our arms are going to be in this goal post series squeeze

those shoulder blades back behind you so we're going to do a little twist so I'm going to take my left arm and I'm going to bring it all the way across to my right hand hello right notice that my legs and my hips are still forward so the action is happening right at the ribs and then I'm going to open that up and then I'm going to bring that other arm across and open it up so don't bring the right arm forward make the left arm come all the way back and open let's do that again remember

the arm comes across don't bring that opposite arm forward and Center let's do it one more time each way are you feeling that movement right into the rib cage I am I I think I'm feeling some pose that we did yesterday or the day before I got a little tightness in my side waist it feels good though one more breath and release don't you like it when you actually feel something in those muscles it's like hmm I think I must have worked those a little bit I like that myself okay so we did this Warrior series

yesterday and we're gonna do it again but we're going to build just a little bit on it okay so we're going to add uh just a couple of things to it but let's start just like we did yesterday so we're going to take this knee and we're going to open it right so our legs are at that 90 degrees we're going to bring those arms up for that Warrior Two pose okay so my ribs are right in the center my head neck and spine are all right in alignment List look over those right fingertips we're going to flip the right palm up to

the ceiling and we're going to take that Palm up and we're going to hold the chair back behind us as we reverse our Warrior now we're going to come back to that Warrior two and then the right arm is going to rest on that right thigh Palm facing up now the hand is in the air let's place it on our waist and lift the heart see how I kind of just lifted and then we're going to extend that on beautiful and let's press back up into that Warrior Two and down we go and let's do the other side just like that so we've done this

one we kind of know it but then then we'll do the little add-on okay so remember you don't ever have to add on right ever ever if this feels better for you you're gonna stay with this version and it's a great version love this version all right we're going to look over our left fingertips now are you in alignment did you check in right making sure let's flip that Palm up we go all the way to the ceiling trying to touch the ceiling then we're going to reverse that Warrior so I'm

looking up if that feels okay on your neck and then we're going to come back down to that Warrior Two and I'm squeezing the muscles against the bones in my arms my upper body is very active here and then I'm going to release and I'm going to Face Forward okay so here's the next little add-on and I'm saying little and I don't mean it's it seems simple but it's a pretty significant stretch additional stretch for those legs oh you know what we didn't do on that side was the side

angle I'll catch it next time I forgot it's okay I'll catch it next time I was so excited about the add-on okay let's come forward in our chair all right so I'm forward now I'm going to take this knee I'm not going to go all the way to 90 degrees okay so I'm just going to do a heel toe and a heel toe so now it's at this diagonal okay now the other leg is going to extend I know how does that feel right so here's a couple of things I want you to think about first thing is

see how I'm up on the side of that foot so I'm not pointing my toe so that I'm dump the toes out my foot is flexed basically and I us up on the edge of that foot do you see what what's going on there so what does that do it changes where the stretch is happening now I'm getting outer and inner thigh stretch do you feel that so here's the other thing if you want to bend the knee a little bit so what will happen in my in-person classes is people will start getting cramps right up in here and I get that so just bend the

knee a little bit and it's fine okay all right are we feeling like we've got that and we're kind of stable on the chair so now I'm going to just go ahead and straighten my leg because it works for me to keep my leg pretty straight I'm feeling quite a bit of stretch on the inner and outer thigh we're going to bring our arms up oh yeah here's a Warrior Two we've got this I'm going to look over my right fingertips and I'm going to flip the right palm to the ceiling I'm going to

take my hand and I'm going to try to touch the ceiling my left hand is going to come down to the chair for a little support I'm lengthening up I'm trying to touch that ceiling then I'm going to come past the midpoint of the body and there's my reverse Warrior I'm looking up if that feels okay on the neck look out if that feels better okay so from here we're going to move to side angle pose I'm not going to forget this time here we go Warrior Two first and now I'm going to put the fleshy part

of that arm my right arm on the fleshy part of that right leg my palm is facing up and I'm lengthening up you see how open my chest is right so I got my wrist my shoulder my shoulder and my are all in in alignment here so I'm not letting myself collapse you've got to really use your abdominals here to make this happen so this looks like if anybody were watching us do this pose they were thinking whatever okay you sit down and do this pose right see what it takes to to be in this position and hold the form

and everything right all right are we ready here we come back up to Warrior Two let's reverse it again we got this back to that Warrior Two squeeze the muscles against the bones and the arms remember if I come in touch try to pull your arm down I couldn't hold it hold it hold it and release ah are you ready to bring that leg in right I know oh take a moment oh it's quite a stretch but it's a good one okay I told you it was an add-on all right here we go let's take this knee we're going to do a heel toe and a heel

toe so remember we've got this angle right here opposite leg extends out now here's the other thing you might find this side is like oh my gosh this one is so much more willing than the other side very common very very common so remember be up on the edge of the foot if you can that's better so we're working the outer thigh here as kind of a Target area for this particular series you can bend that knee a little bit if you need to okay are we ready let's add those arms let's flip that Palm up and back

reversing our Warrior oh my goodness do you feel that I do let's come back to my Warrior Two I'm not going to forget this time okay plus you're part of that left arm comes to the fleshy part of the left leg Palm is facing up so we're going to look up just a little bit if that feels okay or look out but what I do want you to have is that chest is open I know I feel it feel that stretch right we have one more breath here in our side angle pose and up we go into that Warrior Two and let's reverse it one more time

oh yeah and back to that Warrior Two squeeze squeeze squeeze and release oh boy ha okay we're gonna come to standing now and we're gonna be beside our chair and we're gonna do a standing Sun salutation we've done that seated and now we're going to do it in a standing position okay so what I encourage you to do is move forward just a little bit because we're going to be making a circle with our arms and what you don't want to do is hit the back of your chair right does that make sense you've got it

here if you need to hang on to it you can but I'd encourage you to move forward just a little bit so we can make that big so on dive okay so we're gonna reverse one die first so we're going to bring those arms out Palms are facing up we're going to come to our Mountain pose Palms are together overhead and then we're going to bring our hands to our heart really pull your belly in here we're going to keep that belly button to spine nice uh engaged abdominals now we're back to Mountain pose and we're just

going to bring our arms around and we're just going to make that Circle again and bring our hands to Heart okay I just want you to feel that a couple of times before we add on ready let's do that again Palms face up all the way to Mountain pose bring your hands to your heart and then we're going to come back up and we're going to make a big circle with those arms and we're going to come back to heart now we're going to add the breath inhale as we come up to that mountain pose exhale hands to heart I

don't know if you notice but I'm following my hands with my gaze if that feels okay you can do that too inhale up exhale big circle around and bring our hands to our heart okay so now what we're going to add is instead of just making the circle we're going to dive forward all right so you're diving at the hips not at the waist belly stays tight to protect your back ready here we go big circle inhale up Mountain pose exhale bring hands to heart now listen in how we go up exhale we're going to

dive forward all right now we're going to place our hands on our thighs and we're going to extend our head long so head is forward and seat is back this is considered our halfway lift here all right extending nice and long through the spine one more breath we're going to bend our knees and we're going to just roll it up nice and slow okay bring your hands to Heart we're going to do that just like that again inhale up we go Mountain pose exhale hands to heart now if I don't cue the breath you can add

that yoga breath if you want inhale up exhale dive It Forward hands to those thighs extending nice and long into that halfway lip if you want to just breathe normally that's fine too bend the knees roll it up hands to Heart we're going to add a forward fold in up we go hands to Heart back up we go we're gonna die forward use your belly here hands on thighs for a halfway lift now from here I'm just going to let my heart Begin to Fall a little bit forward my hands are still on my thighs for some support there's a

little bit of stretch for those hamstrings let the head fall if that feels okay you can hold the chair bend the knees roll it up and bring your hands to your heart so I want to check in just a minute before we continue if it's making you dizzy you're not going to let your head fall so far right so maybe you're here as you're halfway lived and you just let your head fall a little bit for that forward fold keeping your head above the heart that's fine now if it feels okay and you want to let

that head fall a little bit further that's fine too but I don't want you to feel like you have to do that if it makes you dizzy or if it's just uncomfortable okay you don't have to let's do that again hands to Heart we've only got one more add-on here we go up to Mountain pose let's bring our hands to Heart we're going to come back up to Mountain pose we're going to dive It Forward belly button to spine there we are halfway lift hands on shins I mean thighs extend nice and long forward fold

you've still got your hands on those thighs for support now instead of rolling up what we're going to do is we're going to reverse Swan Dive so my arms are going to go back out there's your back right back is working hard up to Mountain pose bring your hands to your heart we're going to do that again up we go dive It Forward belly button to spine hands on thighs halfway lift inhale exhale let that heart fall forward High reverse Swan Dive up on an inhale Mountain pose bring your hands to your heart we're going to

do that one more time up we go exhale dive It Forward High halfway lift inhale exhale forward fold reverse one dive all the way back up to Mountain pose and bring your hands to your heart how did that feel was that good I love Sun salutation right just get a little bit of movement going get a little bit of flow it's a little vinyasa flow right kind of nice and a little anyway good movement okay so now we are going to do that Warrior Two series again remember we did it yesterday so we're going to do this

one again so we're going to take our foot we're going to place it under the chair remember start with the one next to the back of the chair that's the foot otherwise when you turn it's going to be very confusing okay it's like why don't we do it so this is the leg the left foot and then we're going to take that step back okay hips are forward this is the start of a warrior one We're not gonna do that Warrior one yet we'll do it but for right now we're just gonna turn and move

into that Warrior Two so we're going to bend that front knee and we're kind of our hips are around and we're in that Warrior Two position all right let's look over those front fingertips we're going to flip that Palm up to the ceiling and we're going to reverse our Warrior so I'm looking up if that feels okay on your neck you can always look out if that feels better we're going to come back to that Warrior Two now that hand is just going to come down into the chair and we're going to

open up into that side angle pose and let's go ahead and extend that side angle oh yeah press up into that Warrior Two reverse our Warrior up and back back to Warrior Two and step out of it okay let's do the other side so the leg next to the back of the chair is the one that's going to step under we're going to this other leg is going to step back bring bend that front knee bring the hips around first okay now we're just going to move into that Warrior Two ha where are your ribs right peeking at

the ribs belly is tight looking over those front fingertips let's flip the Palm up and reverse that Warrior up and back now we're going to come to that Warrior two and go straight to side angle pose High lifting up right making sure those shoulders are in alignment with the wrist let's extend there's that side waist that may be why I'm feeling a little bit my Sideways from yesterday are we ready to press up into that Warrior too let's reverse it one more time back to that Warrior Two squeeze the muscles against the bones in

the arms one more breath and release very good let's come back to ascended how does that feel good feel a little stretch happening a little movement I love it I love it I love it okay so we're gonna take our we're gonna move into a crescent lunge we're going to take our right knee we're going to open it and then we're going to let our left knee fall straight down towards the floor push that foot back a little bit right up on those toes if that feels okay for you now I'm going to look over my front

bent knee I'm going to bring my arms up to go post arms so I'm just squeezing my arm my shoulder blades back behind me and I'm looking up where the ceiling and the wall meet one more breath here let's release that we're going to do that again with one little add-on okay back to goal post arms I'm straightening the back of this kneecap is up towards the ceiling now I'm going to take my hands to the ceiling I'm going to inhale to prepare pull that belly in super tight and I'm going to lean over that

front leg there's your back you feel that stretch one more breath here back up we go bring the hands down release and face forward so if that doesn't feel good on your back one thing you can do is keep the elbows bent okay so if extending those arms long is too much for the back then keep the elbows bent and that's going to reduce that lever length and it'll make it a little bit less stressful make sure you keep your belly tight let's do the other side are we ready okay so that left knee is

opening right knee is falling down towards the mat push the foot back okay so feel this first lifting that heart now let's go to goal post arms squeezing the shoulder blades back behind you looking up slightly just one more breath here feel that stretch let's release that okay now we're going to do that again with that little add-on okay so here we go little it's not little is it it's a significant add-on all right let's go post arms squeeze those shoulder blades back behind you you feel it

here we go fingertips to the ceiling inhale here belly tight extend those arms out over that bent knee there's the back pull that belly in Bend those elbows if that feels better one more breath hands to the ceiling oh yeah and down we go go ahead and face forward ah let's sit back in our chair let's place our hands lightly on our thighs flipping the Palms up to the ceiling we're moving into shavasana pose our resting pose close the eyes take a deep breath in and a full breath out pointing towards purpose

Delight in dreaming about what could be but don't take permanent refuge in those unfulfilled dreams instead start working your way to them little by little begin to transform those dreams and your actual reality give yourself credit for everything you've already been able to achieve then point that process of achievement directly at the dreams you long to reach there is Great Value in moving towards something positive and desirable even if you are not fully committed or confident you can go through the motions

and that has value too you are at your best when you are pointing toward a meaningful purpose that purpose will bring energy resourcefulness and determination to the surface go ahead imagine the future in a positive way and take a step in the direction of that future discover for yourself how a positive vision for the future can improve your experience of life right now take a deep breath in and a full breath out drop your right ear towards your right shoulder reach up with the right hand give the head a gentle tug as you press that opposite hand down towards the floor release it drop your chin towards your chest reach up with your hands give the head a gentle tug release it drop your left ear towards your left shoulder reach up with your left hand give the head a gentle tug pressing that right hand down towards the floor release it look out just slightly open your mouth if you want to stretch your jaw bring your hands to your heart honoring one another we say namaste ah very well done my fellow bottoms down these we've made it to the end of day 11. let's just keep showing up and make sure that we come to our chair every day

DAY 12

I'm glad you've joined me today today is day 12 of our 28 day chair yoga journey together now we're going to start seated and then we'll move into standing for more Warrior poses and then we'll move back into our seated position we are going to be using a block today if you have a block that's great if you don't have a block you can substitute a big book or you can just do it without it that's fine too now if you like the experience that you have today I hope you'll click the Subscribe button it's free and leave me a comment I love to hear from you guys so let's get started we're going to sit up nice and tall in our chair we're going to move forward we're not leaning back we're going to take a moment as we focus on that mind and body and breath grounding our feet to the Earth grounding our sits buns to the chair lifting your heart lowering the shoulders out of the ears hands are resting lightly on the thighs

flipping the Palms up to the ceiling closing the eyes and connecting to our breath just feel your natural inhalation and exhalation let's begin to elongate the breath inhaling a little more deeply exhaling a little more completely inhaling a little more deeply exhaling a little more completely one more time inhale and exhale bring your hands to your heart

set your intentions for today's practice one more breath here bring the hands back down to the thighs and Open the Eyes let's drop our right ear towards our right shoulder and drop our chin towards our chest let's drop our left ear towards our left shoulder and chanted chest look forward moving on we're going to do some shoulder rolls now we're going to roll those shoulders forward and up and back and down and we're going to do that again forward up back and down and then we're going to reverse

that ah you know if you can move your head a little bit if you want to in this one roll that neck just a little bit all right very very good okay Mountain pose hands down spread those fingers gold post arms squeeze those shoulder blades behind now we're going to lengthen those hands to the ceiling we're going to bring our palms together interlace your fingers pointer finger is up towards the ceiling and we're going to lean our Mountain and we're going to come up and we're going to lean our Mountain the other way and we're going to come up and we're going to lean again and then we're going to turn and look up at the ceiling take that twist out back up to the ceiling we go and then we're going to lean the other way and we're going to turn and we're going to look up at that ceiling just a little maybe twist take the twist out come back up and bring those hands back down to your lap okay let's do our cat Cow we're going to take our thumbs to the back wall we're going to open up through that chest feel

that openness in the CH in the throat as well right looking up just a little bit and then come down into that catch pose just a couple more inhale up and exhale down we're going to do that again inhale up and exhale down bringing our hands to our heart getting ready for our sun salutation reverse one dive up we go Mountain piles and bring our hands to our heart we're going to come back up to that mountain pose and we're going to Swan Dive forward into that forward salute with airplane arms and we're

going to stretch through that spine and we're going to bring our hands to our tour and let's do that again big circle up we go belly is tight all the way to Mountain pose bring your hands to Heart let's come back up to Mountain pose and dive forward forward salute airplane arms we're going to stretch through that spine nice and long bring those hands to Heart we're going to do that again here we go and up with our Mountain pose bring your hands to heart I'm following my hands with my gaze I'm adding that breath

inhale here exhale we're diving forward forward salute airplane arms now we're going to move to that supported forward fold let the forearms rest on the thighs let the heart fall forward oh yeah there's the back and Tuck that chin and roll it up bring your hands to your heart let's do it big circle up we go Mountain pose bring your hands to heart back up we go to Mountain pose dive it forward forward salute airplane arms that's your exhale inhale to prepare exhale forward fold and roll it up we're gonna add on hands

to Heart let's do it big circle up Mountain pose bring your hands to heart back up to Mountain dive it forward forward salute our plane arms stretch it out forward fold let that heart fall forward pull that belly in Reverse Swan die bring those arms out and up Mountain pose bring your hands to Heart we're going to do that two more times up we go dive It Forward add that breath if you wish forward salute stretch it out forward fold let that heart fall Ready reverse Swan die bring the arms out and around there's your back working up to

Mountain pose bring your hands to Heart last time through we've got this up we go dive it forward forward salute airplane arms let's do that forward fold and reverse Swan dime all the way back up to Mountain pose and bring your hands to our heart how did that feel a little movement right get that blood flowing it was very good so I know we've done that Warrior series we're going to do two things differently we're going to add in a warrior one and then we're also going to um add just a little different leg

position and so we're going to see how we feel on those but we're going to start with our Warrior Two so we're going to do go ahead and move this knee out at that 90 degree angle okay so this is we're building in on that series just a little bit here so Warrior Two to start with looking over those front fingertips right now to move to Warrior one it's a little funky so I'm just going to let you if it feels okay you're gonna do it so all I'm going to do is I'm going to let this

knee fall down towards the mat as I bring that arm up and around you see what I did there so now this knee is straight down towards the floor my arms are up my shoulders are down out of my ears my belly is tight and then I'm going to move back to that Warrior Two let's do that again just like that just to kind of get the feeling of it down that arm goes up to the ceiling there's that lower here one and then I'm going to move back to that Warrior Two do you see what's happening that knee is just kind of falling down

and coming up one more time down we go hands to the ceiling there's your Warrior one and then we're going to move back to that Warrior Two now we're going to move to side angle we've done this one before right we know this one Palm faces up extend that upper arm and then let's go ahead and extend that side angle now we're going to press back into that Warrior Two reverse thy Warrior up and back we're going to go back to Warrior Two and we're going to bring our hands down and we're going to release so how did

that feel so I know that Warrior One Warrior Two to Warrior one is a little funky with the legs but see if that feels okay I like it I mean I think we can do it it's just a little weird Okay so we're going to take this right uh left knee excuse me and open it we've already done the other side haven't we so I've got this 90 degrees to begin with right and let's come up to Warrior Two we've done this when we know this one we feel pretty good with it okay so now what I'm going to do is this

knee is going to fall down towards the mat as I bring this arm down and around and now I'm at my warrior one okay so knee is down towards the floor this leg is still this leg kind of stays where it is it doesn't really move my arms are up to the ceiling does that feel okay stretching him out of here you feel it okay now my outside arm my right arm that's what I'm going to Windmill around and I'm going to come back to Warrior Two okay we ready let's do it again Warrior one and Warrior Two

Warrior one and Warrior Two One More Time Warrior one to Warrior Two let's go to our side angle pose we're going to extend our side angle pose we're going to come back up to Warrior Two let's reverse that Warrior up and back we're going to come back to that Warrior Two and we're going to release okay so let's face forward ha so we did this one yesterday where we added a little extra for the legs so this one we're going to do that one first and then we're going to add one more that's a little even a little

deeper stretch for those inner thighs but let's do the the one we did yesterday first okay so I'm going to take my right knee and I'm going to do a heel toe and a heel toe so my hip my knee and my ankle are in alignment and a little bit of a diagonal I'm a little forward in my chair right so you want to be a little forward and then I'm going to extend the left leg out and I'm up on the edge of that foot remember that and remember that you can bend the knee if you want to it's okay

okay how's that feel right let's come up now to get to that Warrior one from here it's it's even a little more funky but it's okay so we're going to start with this hand we're going to bring it down and around and then we're going to bring our hands up so again I'm going to leave this leg where it is okay so it's a little a little bit of a stretch for here and then I'm going to come back to that Warrior Two let's bring that hand down and around into that Warrior one

and then we're going to move to that Warrior Two and we're going to do that one more time ready down and around to Warrior one and then move to Warrior Two let's come to side angle lifting up through that heart let's extend that side angle looking up at that feels okay on your neck come back to that Warrior Two let's reverse our Warrior up and back back to Warrior Two and release okay ha how'd that feel okay so we're gonna do the other side so let's do it here we go a heel toe and a

heel toe so I'm out of that diagonal extend that right leg out remember try to be up on the side of that foot bend the knee if that feels better for you okay are we ready are the ribs right in the center I kind of felt like my ribs were forward so I brought my ribs back arms out look over those front fingertips flip that Palm up and I don't think I did that on the other side that's okay we're going to reverse our Warrior to start with because I'm making it up as a girl there we go Warrior Two okay now starting with

this backhand we're gonna windmill around to that Warrior one and then we're going to bring that arm back and around to the Warrior Two shoulders are down out of the ears squeeze the muscles against the bones in those arms bring that arm down and around to Warrior one and move back to that Warrior too one more time down we go Warrior one and Warrior Two side angle pose we got it feel that stretch bring that arm by by I call it bicep by ear one more breath pressing up into that Warrior Two and release okay

so we just have one more thing and here's the final piece of that whole series so I'm going to scoot back in my chair so that the seat of my chair is between my legs this leg is going to pretty much stay right where it is and then I'm going to extend this leg out I know right remember you got versions the version where your legs are at 90 degrees and the version we just did where we're forwarding our chair if this doesn't work for you you're going to do one of those other two versions okay we just hang it here for a moment

let's come to that Warrior Two we'll look over those front fingertips we're going to bring that arm down and around into that Warrior one and then we're going to move to that Warrior Two left hand down and around to the ceiling for warrior one and back to Warrior Two one more time down and around the Warrior One move to that Warrior two are we ready side angle pose we've got this lifting up add the extension if you like you don't have to it's just an option back up we go reverse that Warrior

back to Warrior Two and release oh how'd that feel okay we're gonna do the other side so again I'm moving back the seat of my chair is between my legs this knee is pretty much going to stay where it is right so it's already at that diagonal the opposite leg is going to extend I know I feel it too quite the stretch here up on that side of that foot okay are we ready here we go Warrior Two looking over those front fingertips now starting with your right hand you're going to Windmill down and around into

that Warrior one and then you're going to move to your Warrior Two let's do that again dining around to Warrior one and a round to Warrior two one more time and if you don't like the Warrior One funkiness then just stay in Warrior Two Warrior Two side angle puffs I had to make an adjustment there we go and then extend press back to that Warrior Two reverse up and back back to Warrior Two and three release all right Face Forward oh let's give those legs just a moment here actually let's do a little internal

rotation that should feel pretty good ha so all I've done is I've just kind of wrapped my feet are wide and I'm letting my knees fall in towards one another just to kind of counter all of that other external rotation we just did it's just a little internal rotation for those legs one more breath here all right so we're going to come up to standing and we're going to be on the right side of our chair okay now we've done this one before with the Warrior Two we're going to add in that

Warrior one so kind of the same thing we just did seated we're going to add in that Warrior One pose so again the leg next to the seat of the chair I'm just going to move my block just a little bit the leg next to the seat of the chair is the one that we're going to start with okay so we're going to bend that knee and the opposite leg is going to step back hips are forward now from this position what I want you to think about is pulling your belly in super tight right so pulling that belly in and lengthening through that tailbone

so I want you to feel like your weight is coming back so holding the chair is fine standing down that back leg weight is back bend the front knee okay bring your hands to Heart all right inhale here and then exhale extend the arms up to the ceiling for our Warrior One pose now starting with this right hand the outside hand we're going to Windmill around to that Warrior Two my front knee is still bent okay we're going to flip that front Palm up and back for that reverse Warrior then we're going to come down and we're

going to put that hand in the chair for our side angle pose then we're going to bring our bicep by our ear for that extended side angle pose press up to that Warrior Two flip the Palm up and back back to Warrior Two shoulders down belly tight Ribs Right in the center of the body and release okay very good let's do the other side so see how adding that Warrior one actually um kind of makes it easier to get into Warrior too I think so that was a nice little addition so we're going to bend that front knee so I want to when you

bend it you're touching right so you're able to touch the chair so that's just going to help you when you come into side angle to know that that chair is in the right position okay so now my hips are going to come forward facing the chair they want to be at a diagonal but I want you to see if you can bring them all the way around bend that front knee standing down that back leg so remember belly tight extending nice and long through the spine bring the hands to the heart and then extend those arms up

for your one okay are we ready to move to Warrior Two so I'm just windmilling those arms around my knee is still touching the chair I'm looking over my right fingertips flip the Palm up and back reversing my warrior back to Warrior two and then that right hand is going to come into the chair for side angle pose extending nice and long opening through the chest arm extends over if you like that press back up into Warrior Two reverse the Warrior One More Time back to Warrior Two and release okay very very good now

let's come back to the other side of our chair and we're going to do a pyramid pose if you don't have a block it's fine you're just going to use your chair and then if you want a little deeper you're going to use your leg but since I have a block I'm just going to go ahead and use it I uh it's just going to help me out a little bit so to bring that block on the we call this the number three position the tallest position and I'm going to place it right there in my chair and my

foot's going to go beside it okay now for Pyramid pose this front leg unlike with our Warrior series where the knee was bent now that leg is going to stay straight okay but the back leg is still going to step back and that foot's going to be at that 45 degree angle so the heel is down we're going to bring those hips around so that one of the really important pieces of this pose is keeping this hip back so the hip of the leg that's long that's extended that's straight in front of you that's the one

that's always going to want to come around so just think about keeping that hip back you might even grab your thumb and bring it right here to the hip crease to remind you okay all right so the first thing we're going to do is we extend long through the spine pull the belly in right hinging at the hips we're going to keep the back flat as we come forward place your hands in the seat of the chair and see if you can let the heart come forward anymore you feel the stretch in that leg right so the stretch is happening in the back

side of the front leg so I'm just kind of bending those elbows letting my heart fall keep this hip back right feel that one more breath here and we're going to go ahead and come up now we're going to stay on this side and do two more add-ons and then we'll go to the other side okay so we're going to stay on this side for now so remember keep that hip back lengthen through the spine now this time as I come forward I'm going to place my hand on my block instead of my chair so maybe that gives me a little deeper

stretch maybe your hands are if you don't have the block your hands are on your leg which is fine keep that hip back do not let that um this hip of the leg that's extended don't let it come forward letting that heart fall one more breath here okay let's bend the front knee as we roll up grab your chair okay how did that feel so now I'm going to move my block down and we'll see how that works alright so here we go hip back hinge forward maybe your hands are in the seat of the chair maybe your hands are on your leg

maybe your hands are on your block just a little deeper into that triangle pose we have one more breath bend the knee and come up okay we have one final piece now this is pretty significant so I want you to only do it if it feels okay but instead of our hands coming down to our block we're going to have our hands behind our back ah there's going to be a little balance work here so keep your belly tight clasp your hands behind your back lift up through the heart right squeezing those shoulder blades behind now pull that

belly in as you begin to let your heart fall forward your hands are going to come up behind you and just as you know whatever works for you one more breath here let's release the hands to the chair bend the knee come up to a standing position how did that feel okay we're going to do the other side so I like just doing all three of these uh this series on the same leg because we're just getting a little deeper into the stretch right so first thing I want to do is just set my block here give myself that option

okay so my front leg again I want the foot to be under the chair so you've got the chair right in close enough proximity that you can grab it if you need it my hips are forward I'm staying that back leg is straight and my heel is down okay so turn those hips forward remember if you want to grab the the where the crease of the leg and the hip are and pull that hip back just think about that we want to keep this hip back nice long through the spine just begin to let your heart fall forward place your hands on

that chair and maybe you bend the elbows a little bit it doesn't matter right if that doesn't work ah pyramid pose okay let's bend the knee and roll up okay now we're going to do it again this time my hands are going to go to my block so let's hinge forward maybe the hands are on the leg maybe the hands are on the Block just getting a little deeper into that stretch right one more breath okay bend the knee and come up I'm going to move my block down are we ready nice long spine belly tight

hinge forward keep this leg straight keep the hip back hinge down we go one more breath bend that knee up we go okay you want to do the final version let's do it clasp your hands behind your back push those Knuckles down squeeze your shoulder blades back are we ready belly tight we're going to calm down oh we're bowing over that front leg our hands are coming up behind us so that upper back or our shoulders are getting a nice stretch in addition to that front leg we have three and two and one grab the chair bend that knee

roll it up into standing excellent work let's come back into seated okay so we're going to take our right knee and we're going to open it nice and wide and let our left knee fall down towards the floor move back into that Crescent lunge so back of the kneecap towards the ceiling nice stretch for the front side of that leg holding onto the chair or to your front thigh let's release it and we're going to do that again and face forward okay let's extend that leg out in front of us toes to the

ceiling lengthen through the spine let the heart fall forward keeping the back flat looking out Beyond those toes and roll it up and let's do that again nice long spine inhale to prepare exhale let that heart and up we go so we're going to move into pigeon pose you can cross at the ankle right so this is great you can just cross right here at the ankle or you can extend your right leg and cross your left ankle onto that shin it's a great version and then the final version if you so desire is going to be ankle to knee so

I'm going to let you pick which of those three versions you prefer I'm going to stay with this version everybody whichever version your legs are in you're going to extend your spine nice and long and let your heart begin to fall forward oh yeah feeling that stretch let's tuck our chin and roll up we're just going to move that knee up and down a little bit I call that fluttering the butterfly wing let's extend through the spine keeping the back flat let that heart fall forward tuck in that chin and rolling it up all

right let's unravel go to the other side left knee opens 90 degrees let the right knee fall down towards the floor push the foot back lift the heart up feel that stretch bless your release and we're going to do that again back of the kneecap towards the ceiling lifting up through the heart and release let's go ahead and face forward we're going to extend that right leg long okay toes are to the ceiling lengthen nice and long through the spine pyramid pose letting the heart fall forward keeping the back flat looking out beyond

your toes tuck the chin and roll it up and let's do that again nice long spine inhale to prepare exhale down we go one more breath and up we go remember you can cross at the ankle if you like that better you can cross at the shin or you can cross at the knee pigeon pose you can choose all right are we ready last long spine whichever version your legs are in let's all lengthen through the spine keep the back flat as we begin to let that heart fall forward feeling the stretch right hearing that glute area let's tuck that chin and roll

it up and then we're going to do that again nice long through the spine inhale and then exhale we're going to come forward and then up we go okay unravel those legs let's move back in our chair you can lean back hands are resting lightly on the thighs flip the Palms up take a deep breath in and out let's do that again take a deep breath in and then as you exhale let those eyes close or soften you are the person you are the person who does the difficult thing because it is the right thing

the world moves forward because of what you do you are the person who looks for ways to embrace responsibility instead of searching for places to cast blame by doing so you transform problems into opportunities defeat into victory you are the person who seeks to understand when so many others are merely shouting empty platitudes you are the person who cares enough to listen who listens enough to care even more it's not easy to do what you do to be who you are but you know that some things are more important than merely making the easiest

choice you are the person who does not seek praise but who would like to know every now and then that you're appreciated so look around see life being lived and know that life itself appreciates what you do more than any one person could ever realize you are the person who makes a difference whenever you have the opportunity to do so you live as if your life matters and it most certainly does take a deep breath in and a full breath out take a deep breath in and out drop your right ear towards your right

shoulder reach up with the right hand give the head a gentle tug as you press that left hand down towards the floor release it drop your chin towards your chest reach up with your hands give the head a gentle tug release it drop your left ear towards your left shoulder reach up with the left hand give the head a gentle tug pressing that right hand down towards the floor release it look up just slightly open your mouth if you want to stretch your jaw bring your hands to your heart

DAY 13

let's get started so we're going to start by sitting up nice and tall in our chair we're moving forward we're going to connect that mind body and breath both of our feet are on the floor and we're grounding each foot to that Earth and we're going to ground those sits bones to our chair so feeling like you're not leaning one way or the other we're going to lift our heart up nice and Tall pull those shoulders down out of our ears place our hands lightly on the thighs Palms face up close your eyes and connect to that breath drawing your attention inward towards the Heart Center letting go of everything outside of the room we're going to move that breath down into the diaphragm as we inhale the belly extends we're filling our lungs from the bottom up and as we exhale actively pulling the belly button in towards the spine pushing the air up and out of the lung so do that a couple of times and breathe normally we're going to do that again we're going to inhale to four counts with our diaphragmatic breath and we'll exhale to five it'll be something like this inhale two three four exhale two three four five inhale two three four exhale two

three four five and breathe normally bring your hands to your heart set your intentions for today's practice one more breath here bring your hands back down to your thighs and open your eyes we're going to roll our shoulders just a little bit here nice little openness for those shoulders right and then reverse it I like to move my head around a little bit too very nice let's move into our Mountain pose spread those fingers wide nice long spot extending those arms up to the ceiling Palms together interlace fingers pointer

finger to the ceiling and we're going to lean our Mountain and we're going to come up and we're going to lean our Mountain the other way and we're going to come up we're going to bring those hands back down spread those fingers wide extend that mountain up belly button to spine lengthen interlace fingers Point your finger to the ceiling and we're going to lean our Mountain and we're going to come up and we're going to lean or Mountain the other way and we're going to come up and we're

going to bring our hands down spread those fingers out back up we go Mountain pose Palms together pointer finger to the ceiling we're going to lean our mountain and we're going to twist take a little baby twist look to the ceiling take the twist out come up other side lean lift twist look up at the ceiling take the twist out back up we go bring those hands down and roll those shoulders again oh yeah maybe you wrote them one at a time and let's reverse it bring your hands to your heart nice long spine lifting up open through the chin

pull those ribs back moving into cow pose thumbs to the back wall lifting up nice and long through the spine looking up slightly hands to thighs round down into cat warming up that spine a little bit let's come back into cow pose again thumbs to the back wall we lift up through the heart looking up slightly and down into Pat's pose inhale up into cow we go exhale down into cats we go last time inhale into cow and exhale into our cat pose hold and breathe one more breath and release very very good okay we're going to bring our hands

to Heart now we're going to make a big circle around up into our Mountain pose and we're going to bring those hands to Heart moving into our little Sun salutation series here a little warm up we're going to dive forward into that forward salute with airplane arms we're going to stretch through that spine moving to that forward fold let that heart fall we're supporting with our hands on those thighs tuck the chin and roll it up bring your hands to your heart big circle up we go into that mountain pose and we bring our hands to

our heart we're going to come back up to Mountain and we're going to dive forward forward salute airplane arms remember stretching through that spine nice and long let's do that forward fold we're supporting with our arms on our thighs giving that a little bit of support for that upper body tuck the chin roll it up bring your hands to your heart last time through big circle up we go Mountain pose bring your hands to your heart we're coming back to Mountain pose and we're gonna dive forward forward salute

airplane arms stretch it out forward fold let that heart fall forward oh yeah tuck the chin and rolled it up into a seated position okay very very good A little bit of warm up there we're ready to move on to our next pose okay so we're going to do a seated Eagle pose now so we're going to start by just crossing ankle to ankle okay we've got our ankles crossed at one ankle on top of the other okay now we're going to bring our wrists and we're going to cross wrist to wrist we're going to twist to the right

and we're going to come Center and we're going to twist to the left and we're going to come Center we're going to bring our arms up towards the ceiling as we look up and center and then we're going to bring those arms down as we look down towards our lap and then we're going to come up and we're going to unravel and unravel and let's go to the other side okay so as you cross your ankle to ankle leave your left leg where it is make your right leg crossover okay so I'm not bringing this foot in I'm going to make

my right leg cross all the way over endless cross wrist to rest okay are we ready we're going to twist to the left first and then Center to the right and Center up Center down Center and release okay so that's a great version and if you want to stick with that version you're going to stick with that version but if you want to add on what I'm going to do now is instead of Crossing ankle to ankle I'm going to cross my leg over okay so again if that doesn't feel good for you you're going to stick with the at the previous

version and that's fine okay so the LA the second thing you can do is you can stick with that wrist to wrist okay if you want to do a little bit more what I'm going to do is I'm going to open my arms nice and wide I'm going to take my left arm on top and I'm going to hug myself okay is that feeling alright can you lift your elbows up just a little all right here we go we're going to twist to the right and we're going to come Center and we're going to twist to the left and we're going to come Center

elbows up and Center and elbows down and Center okay let's unravel and let's unravel those legs okay now we're going to cross the other leg on top we're going to bring those arms out wide now this time the right arm is going to go on top okay so hug yourself right arm top Let's Twist to the left Center twist to the right Center elbows up Center elbows down and center and unravel and unravel okay that feel okay excellent okay so we're going to take our right knee and we're going to open

it up and then we're going to bring our left knee and bring it around so now I'm facing the side wall okay you got that so both knees are facing towards the the side wall now I'm going to bring my hands up to the ceiling my shoulders stay down my belly stays tight now this outside arm is the one I'm going to start with and I'm going to Windmill around so that you're facing me checking in making sure those arms are parallel to the mat take this hand bring it down and around all the way back up to ceiling now start

with the other arm and you're going to Windmill and you're going to be looking over the back of your chair and we're going to bring those hands up to the ceiling we're going to come to goal post arms squeeze your shoulder blades back behind you looking up slightly bring their hands back up to the ceiling bring the hands down to your lap and face forward how did that feel pretty good yeah let's do the other side okay so we're going to open up first bring that other knee around now I'm

facing the other wall okay you got it both knees are facing the other wall let's bring those hands up to the ceiling now I'm going to start again with this outside arm right so we're going to Windmill around face to me hello arms to the ceiling start with the other arm windmill around face the back of your chair arms to the ceiling goal post arms squeeze your shoulder blades behind you lift your heart feel a little bit of arch in the back belly tight looking up slightly one more breath here arms back to the

ceiling bring the hands down and release how did that feel yeah I like that one I think that was kind of nice okay we're going to come to standing on the right side of our chair now this is a standing Eagle series and we're going to be doing quite a few different add-ons and remember you don't ever have to add on you can always revert back and do the previous version always okay so just remember that so we're going to take our feet hip distance apart and what I mean by that is it's not you're not too wide but your

feet aren't together so you want to have that stable base so if you look down your hips are in alignment pretty much with those ankles okay so we're going to cross one a wrist to the other wrist belly is tight all right shoulders are down out of the ears now we're going to twist to the right my hips and my knees stay forward Let's Twist Center twist the other way twist Center and release okay now we're going to do the same thing with the other wrist in front Okay so I personally did left in front now

I'm going to do right in front Okay shoulders are down belly tight now we're going to twist over our chair first and they were going to come Center and we're going to twist the other way and Center and release okay so excellent version now the next add-on is we're going to move to those Eagle arms okay so I'm going to bring my arms out to the side now I'm going to bring my right arm on top and I'm going to hug myself I'm going to twist I don't know let's do it over the chair first it doesn't

matter and Center twist the other way and center now listen we're going to go up a little arch in the back I'm looking up Center and then I'm going to take my elbows down towards the floor just a little stretch for that upper back and Center and let's open those arms and now let's cross the other arm on top squeeze hug yourself Let's Twist to the right and we're going to come Center and twist to the left and we're going to come Center elbows up and Center elbows down and center and release okay so those are

really good versions either of those is excellent so the add-on here is a little balance work okay so we're going to lift a knee you're like I don't want to lift my knee so this hold on to that chair to start with and I would encourage you to start putting the weight into the leg next to the chair and lifting that other knee up okay does it really matter but personally I think if I'm going to fall I want you know I just want to have I want to be who I can grab that chair that it doesn't really matter that's my

my thought process anyway okay are we ready now we're gonna not do the eagle arms we're gonna do the crossing wrist to wrist okay all right so remember balance is all about abdominals pulling in tight pelvic floor muscles lift find a spot in front of you that's not moving focus in on that spot are we ready we're going to let go of the chair and we're going to cross wrist to wrist belly tight okay are we ready we're going to twist to the left and we're going to come Center and we're going to twist to the right

and we're going to come Center and down we go how did you do I know I was wiggling everywhere right let's come to the other side there's nothing wrong with that either so that ankle wrote you know wobbling back and forth is fine it's basically just the brain and the leg talking so it's okay so don't think oh my gosh I'm doing something wrong you're not okay are we ready we're gonna put the weight into that leg next to the chair and let's bring that other knee up it's a little table top leg so remember

belly in pull the and I'll tell you right now this side could be more willing or less swelling generally speaking we have one side that's more willing to do these balance poses than the other super common okay so belly's super tight pelvic floor muscles lift we get our core engaged right shoulders are down now if you'll find a spot that's not moving in front of you and focus in on that spot it helps we're going to cross wrist to wrist let's turn and face our chair walk right belly tight Carol let's turn and face

our chair so the dynamic movement here is super challenging too we're going to come Center we're going to go the other way and we're going to come Center and we're going to put that foot down behindfully how did you do I love a little bit of balance just a little bit right excellent work okay let's come back to the right side of our chair now we're going to turn and face our chair we're going to work into a little bit of forward fold now I think we've done a little four we're filming I remember I think we've done some forward folding but we're just going to build into it a little deeper it's okay right it's all good so this one is again you want to really keep your abdominals tight because what that does is that protects that back okay so here we go I'm going to take a little step away from my chair this is not balanced so you can hold on to that chair pull that belly in that's nice and tight now I'm going to bend right here at the hinge right at the hips slowly folding forward and I'm going to

place my hands in the seat of the chair and I'm going to bring my weight just a little bit forward now I'll tell you if this really bothers your wrists you can come into fists so that keeps those wrists straight instead of bending at the wrist okay so that's always an option anytime we have our hands in the seat of the chair okay so I'm going to go ahead and flatten mine my wrists are okay so I'm going to go ahead and flatten my wrists my Palms if you will now I'm going to bend my elbows and

begin to let my heart fall how does that feel right so don't worry about how far down you come it doesn't matter what I would rather you concentrate on is keeping the legs straight micro Bend to the knee is fine but don't start bending the knees we want to stretch those hamstrings so the minute you bend the knees you're disengaging the hamstring stretch okay so let's keep those legs straight let's begin to let that heart fall forward so for me personally I've got my forehead resting on the seat of my chair

I'm not saying that you need to do that I'm just saying that if that works for you that is a a great version of this forward mode you feel very supported belly is tight one more breath okay well I'm going to bend my knees pretty generously and I'm going to roll up into a standing position okay so remember anytime we're going to do that one more time anytime we get our head below our heart if it makes you dizzy then I encourage you not to take the head so far down okay you don't have to but for me it feels fine and so I kind of let my head go down below my heart and I get into an inversion which is a nice thing to do in your yoga practice if it works for you okay we're going to do that one more time all right are we ready I'm going to bend right here hinge at the hips I want to put my hands in the seat of the chair I'm going to bring my weight just a little bit forward then I'm going again to bend my elbows and then maybe my forehead touches maybe it doesn't my legs are straight I'm feeling the back side of the body stretching and my forward fold in three two one bend the knees generously and roll it all the way back up to standing okay now we're gonna add one little thing to that forward fold and what what is called is a straddle forward fold so now I'm going to take my feet wide so at least the width of the chair legs preferably even a little bit more if that feels okay for you okay so we're going to go back to that forward fold so I'm going to hinge right here at the hips I'm going to bring my heart forward my hands in the chair and

I'm going to bring my weight forward okay just like we did a minute ago if you want to let your heart fall a little bit further go for it don't put your forehead down though and you'll see why here in just a second all right are we ready we're going to bend that right knee you're going to feel the inner thigh stretching on that left leg then we're going to come up and we're going to bend the other knee and feel that inner thigh stretching on the other side and then we're going to come up and then

I want you to just roll up into standing and check in and see how that felt okay so we're going to do that again and I encourage you to think about pushing your hips back so we don't want the knees to come forward so as we hinge we want the hips to go back okay so you kind of see what I'm doing there all right let's go ahead and do this again so let's go ahead and hinge down put your hands into the seat of the chair all right so actually for me it's almost like my forearms are down now if that

feels okay go for it whatever feels good for you it's it's fine whichever version okay so now I'm going to bend my left knee and there's the inner thigh stretching on that right side oh my goodness do you feel that let's come up and we're going to bend our other knee so do you notice how I'm pushing my hips back and up we go let's do that again come up and we're going to be in that right knee okay now we're going to come up now the last little piece of this what we're

going to do is it's called revolving and it's just adding a Twist okay so my hands are in the chair I'm going to bend my right knee oops I'm going to bend my right knee to start with then I want you to take your right hand and you're going to open do you see what I'm doing there oh yeah revolving my uh straddle forward fold now we're going to bring that hand back down to the chair and we're going to straighten that leg now I'm going to bend my left knee and I'm going to open that left arm up revolving bring that hand back down to the chair straighten the legs we're going to do that one more time on each side bending that right knee right arm opens up make sure this knee is behind those toes shooting those hips back feeling that stretch and down we go straighten that leg now bend your left knee and open up the other side one more breath here bring the hand back down to the chair straighten both legs heel toe those feet back together and roll up into standing hi let's come to seated how did that feel right I love that one

it was so good all right so we're going to let our right knee we're going to open it up let the left knee fall down Crescent lunge push the foot back lift the heart let's release it and do that again and face forward let's do the other side we're going to open it up let this knee fall down push the foot back lift that heart I'm going to stretch for that front side of that leg right and release it one more time and release facing forward let's just do a little pigeon pose here remember you

can do the ankle to ankle version if you like that one better or you can do ankle to knee we're going to lengthen through the spine and let that heart fall forward should feel pretty good oh man yeah let's go ahead and roll it up and now we're going to do that again nice long spine and then I'm just going to push gently on this leg just get a little bit more if you don't have to right just an add-on don't do it if you don't want it's okay and roll it up okay let's do the other

leg lengthen nice and long through the spine let that heart fall forward keeping the back flat looking out not down you got it and up we go let's do that one more time nice long spine let that heart pop forward pressing gently if you wish one more breath and release oh very good let's sit back getting ready for shavasana bows haha hands resting lightly on those thighs flip the Palms up to the ceiling nice long spine take a deep breath in and out go ahead and close those eyes work to achieve

don't ask yourself what you want to achieve ask yourself what you want to work to achieve it's not enough to have the desire for a particular outcome you must also have the desire to do whatever is necessary to create that outcome it's easy to imagine yourself enjoying the reward it's more challenging to Envision yourself doing the difficult and tedious work necessary to earn that reward yet the people who earn the most coveted rewards not only Envision the necessary work they see it through to completion

achievement often looks easy and glamorous from the outside because all you usually see is the completed job you're the one doing the achieving it's a whole lot of work so be willing to do that work and you'll be the one doing the achieving which is a very good place to be take a deep breath in and a full breath out drop your right ear towards your right shoulder reach up with the right hand give the head a gentle tug pressing that left hand down towards the floor release it drop your chin towards your chest

reach up with the hands give the head a gentle tug release it drop your left ear towards your left shoulder reach up with the left hand give the head a gentle tug pressing that right hand down towards the floor release it look up just slightly open your mouth if you want to stretch your jaw bring your hands to your heart honoring one another we say namaste ha very well done my fellow bottoms down knees we've made it to the end of day 13.

DAY 14

I'm so glad you've joined ume today so today is day 14 of our 28 day Journey we are halfway through it's going so fast okay so we're gonna take a little rest today do a few relaxing poses both seated and standing now we're going to be using the block today and you know if you don't have that block don't worry about it you can use a big book if you have a big book or you can just do it without it it'll be fine and you know I'm going to set my block back behind it just kind of feels good I'm going to lean up against that block for this beginning position or beginning set of poses whatever all right and remember if you like what you're experiencing here I hope you'll click that subscribe button and it is free and I really do enjoy hearing from you guys so leave me a comment okay let's get started so we're going to sit up nice and tall and if you want to lean back against your block for support go for it we're connecting we're going to connect

that body mind and breath so let's take our feet to the floor and sits bones are equally weighted our spine is nice and long our shoulders are down out of the ears we know the drill right hands are resting lightly on the thighs flip the Palms up close your eyes then connect to that breath now with every inhalation just think about lengthening through the spine spine and then exhale and then on that next inhalation see if you can lengthen that spine any longer and then exhale let's do that again inhale and exhale

one more nice long spine inhale and exhale exhale bring your hands to your heart set your intentions for today's practice focusing in on what you want to accomplish bring your hands back down to our thighs and open your eyes so we're going to do another breathing exercise today we're going to place our hands right here at our ribs so you've got one hand on each side of the ribs now I want you to inhale and see if you can feel the ribs expanding out and then exhale see if you can bring those ribs back Center let's

do that again inhale and exhale do that again inhale and exhale and then just release that and take a note just a few normal breaths so sometimes when we're breathing like that we can get a little like light-headed and so we just want to take a couple of normal breaths in between and now we're going to take one hand to our belly and the other hand to our back and we're going to do that same thing so as you breathe see if you can feel the the rib cage and expanding front and back okay let's do that inhale

and exhale front and back body expands inhale and exhale let's do that one more time inhale and exhale and then just breathe normally okay so now we're going to try we're not going to hold our hands and hold anything but I want you to just visualize the side and the front and back so the whole rib cage is filling with air and then releasing let's do that here we go inhale and exhale notice how my belly extends inhale and exhale just one more inhale and exhale and release so just a little mindful breathing there should feel pretty good

okay so the next one is a little bit it's called Head nods and this is gonna you're gonna feel a little stretch in the upper back and the neck so we're going to start with our hands on our knees Palms are facing down now you're going to let your head fall down just like we were going to do a capped pose okay so I'm tucking my chin and I'm letting my head fall looking down at my lap from here I want you to squeeze your shoulder blades behind you so what will happen is your hands position is going

to move from the knees up towards the thighs so I'm squeezing my shoulder blades behind me my hand position has moved now you're just simply going to let your hands float up off of your legs and I want you to bounce your hands up and down actually I should say the arms so the wrists are not flapping the arm is one unit and we're just bouncing those arms up and down up and down up and down bring the hands down to the lap release the shoulder blades and let go let just let your head come up okay we're going to do that again did you

kind of feel what was happening there all right let's try it again hands are going to be on the thighs pawns facing on the knees Palms facing down tuck the chin and let the head fall like a little cat pose here now from here leave your head down your chin is tucked we're going to squeeze our shoulder blades behind us and the hand position is going to move from the knees a little bit forward towards the thighs hold that squeeze behind your shoulders lift your hands up off the mat pulse your arms up and down

pause pause pause three two one and release how did that feel that was quite a stretch for me I feel that one in my neck my upper back I'm just rolling my shoulders a little bit and moving my head a little side to side all right excellent excellent excellent so now we're going to grab our block if you again if you don't have a block don't worry about it it's fine you'll do it without it so I'm gonna put the Block in my right hand and I'm going to bring that right arm kind of like goal post

arms let's bring the other arm up now I want you to bring this arm across and I want you to grab the block and then you're going to open other arm is going to come across and we're going to grab the block and we're going to open let's do that again bring it across grab the block and open and if you don't have the block you're just kind of bringing that arm across and touching right and open let's do one more on both sides here we go open bring it across grab the block and open arm comes across grabs the block

and open and release okay really really good so we're going to take our block and we're going to put it between our feet in that number three position so the tallest position put it right between those feet you're going to take your arms your well let's extend the spine nice and long first we're going into a seated forward fold and we're going to bring our forearms to the thighs Palms facing up and we're going to let our heart fall forward so our supported forward fold let's tuck our chin and roll it up

come up to seated extend the spine nice and long pull the belly button in let that heart fall forward keep the back flat down we go are you looking out not down tuck the chin and roll it up okay so that's version one it is excellent version now if you want to move with me we're going to add on and we're going to put our hands on the Block instead of our hands on our thighs now if you don't have the block what you'll do is you'll walk your hands down your legs okay let's do it extend the spine long

inhale to prepare exhale I'm going to come forward my back is flat I'm going to place my hands on the Block and I'm going to let my heart fall forward tuck the chin and roll it up come up to stand seated extending nice and long through the spine inhale exhale come down hands to that block let that heart fall forward remember if you don't have the block your hands are on your thighs tuck the chin and roll it up okay how's that feel let's work that block down to the number two position so it's this right it's a

little bit lower extend nice and long through the spine on an inhale exhale keep the back flat come down looking out not down hands on that block now we're going to tuck our chin and we're going to roll it up and let's do that again nice long spine on an inhale exhale we're going to go down hands to that block down we go tuck that chin and roll it up and release you know where we're headed let's take that block down to the number one position nice long spine inhale to prepare keep that back flat down we go place the

hands on that block tuck that chin and roll it up are we ready to do that again nice long spine inhale to prepare exhale forward we go hands to that block tuck that chin let the head fall if that feels okay for you roll it back up into a seated position ah okay so now the final piece of this series if you want remember you don't have to because we're going to move that block we're going to take our hands to the floor okay are we ready I'm going to heel toe my feet a little bit wider just so that when I come down I've got a

spot for my belly to hang are you ready nice long spine inhale to repair exhale down we go here we go let's bring those hands to the floor now if you want to tuck your chin and look under your chair there's a nice inversion all right let's roll it up pull that belly in roll it up into a seated position let's do that again nice long spine inhale here exhale down we go hands to the floor tuck the chin let the head fall take two deep breaths in one more breath here we're gonna roll it up into a seated position okay

so if that's feeling alright and you're not getting dizzy and everything's good what we're going to do for the final piece of this is when we're down we're going to take our hands off of the floor we're going to grab our elbows and we're going to hang out in what's called rag doll okay so it's going to be a nice stretch for that back all right are we ready nice long spine inhale exhale down we go hands to the floor let the head fall if that feels okay for you grab your elbows

and now we're hanging out in Ragdoll so you should be feeling more in the back the lower back is stretching do you feel that that's not our head yes Shake our head no not our head yes drop the hands back to the floor pull the belly button in super tight and roll back up into seated position have that for you ah very nice forward fold series so now we're going to do another little stretch for the neck and this one what we're going to do is we're going to bring our hands behind our back okay and then we're going to squeeze our

shoulder blades back together so I'm just I've got my hands clasped behind my back my shoulder blades are back behind I'm squeezing my shoulders are down out of the ears my belly is tight and I'm going to drop my ear to my shoulder oh yeah just a little different neck stretch right okay let's drop our chin towards our chest so try not to lose the squeeze behind that that's kind of what's adding the differentness to this stretch and then we're going to do the other side and then we're going to tuck the chin

and let the head fall one final time release the hands from behind your back lift your head up and let's just do a little shoulder roll because we're going to do that one more time all right ready clasp the hands behind the back push those Knuckles down towards the seat of the chair squeeze your shoulder blades behind you drop your left ear to your left shoulder and Chin to chest let's do the other side one more chin to chest release the hands and release the neck and roll those shoulders oh yeah okay we're gonna thread the needle so

I'm going to take my right hand and we'll place it on my right knee this is the space right here between my arm and my leg that I'm going to thread my other arm through but I'm going to bring that arm up first so I want you to think about stacking one set of ribs on top of the other set of ribs so it's a little twist here now I'm going to bring that ham through Palm is facing up my left ear ear is going to go down towards my left or towards my lap now let's bring that arm up so now my

right ear is kind of towards my lap I'm I'm stacking my rib cage and then I'm going to bring that hand through and then I'm going to thread my needle and now the on the opposite ribs are on top and then we're going to do that one more time up we go thread that hand through one more breath here and release oh that feels so good to me a little stretch through the side waist right okay let's do the other side hand on that thigh opposite arm is going to twist up stacking those ribs let's bring that

hand through Palm faces up all the way through and kind of looking up hand comes up twisting bring the hand through other side one more time up we go hand comes through as we twist looking up and release excellent work let's take that right arm and bring it across our body opposite arm I'm going to kind of Stack one elbow on the other and then I'm bringing pulling in with this opposite arm to get a little stretch so just pull this shoulder down right and then if you want to take a wrist Circle here rotation there if the wrists do for

to go for that and then let's reverse that wrist okay let's release that and we're going to go to the other side so other arm comes across first shoulder down hook right here and then pull there's a nice stretch for that upper arm do a little rotation for the wrist if you like that and reverse it and let's release that oh very very very good okay so we're going to come to standing and we're going to go behind our chair okay so let's go ahead and come up to standing and we're going to come behind our chair so this is a very gentle twist and we'll be we'll be doing one little add-on to our twist to get a little deeper into it but don't you know don't feel like you have to we can stay with the the first twist so I'm going to take my left hand I'm going to bring it right here to the left side of my the chair the other arm is going to come back by my hip I'm going to bend at the elbow just a little bit and I'm going to pull that shoulder back and then I'm going to turn

and I'm going to look over that right shoulder so having your hand on the chair here I can give myself a little leverage but don't let the hips move I want the hips to stay forward and I want the twist to happen at the ribs and let's face forward so now my right arm is going to be on the outside of that chair back my opposite arm Bend at the elbow a little bit pull that shoulder back and then I'm just going to turn and look over the back of it's over that left shoulder I had one more breath and I'm on Face

Forward okay so that that's a great diversion and the only difference we're going to do is instead of the hand being on this this side of the chair is going to come over here it's just going to add a little bit to the twist all right are we ready so now my left hand is on the right side of the chair opposite hand by my hip bend the elbow a little bit pull the shoulder back turn and look make sure those hips do not come with the hips need to stay forward The Twist is happening right at the ribs one more breath face forward and let's

do that on the other side here we go arm is on the hand is on this side of the chair opposite arm back by my hip pull the shoulder back keep the hips forward turn and look over that shoulder and we're hanging out and breathing we have one more breath and face forward excellent so we're going to thread the needle standing now we did it seated we're going to do it standing so I'm going to take a little step back so that I've got some space between the back of my chair and my body so I'm going to take my left arm and I'm

going to rotate up towards the ceiling you're going to bend your right knee okay and we're going to bring that arm up now this hand is going to thread through and then I'm going to bend my other knee as I rotate through and I'm looking up let's do that again bending the opposite knee as that arm comes up and then through it goes and I'm bending the opposite knee and I'm looking up and let's do that one final time so kind of stacking the ribs one on one set on top of the other and then as I come through the opposite set of ribs heads on top and off we go let's do the other side here we go right arm comes up left knee bends up we go now bring through and move through into that thread the needle the opposite knee is bendy and up we go think about stacking those ribs bring that hand through and to the other side last time up we go arm comes through bending the opposite knee and release all right that's very very good so we're going to do our forward fold again and we'll have our block here with us

so let's place that block right on the again on that number three position right between our legs okay pull that chair so I've got a little step back here I'm going to bend hinge right at the hips and I'm going to come forward place the hands in the seat of the chair remember this version we did it yesterday you can bend those elbows and this is a great version of your forward fold let's bend the knees and roll it up into standing okay so now if you want to do a little bit more just if you want you're going to

use the block instead of the seat of the chair so you see how the block is lower right so now I just moved back just a smidge to give myself a little more space I've still got the chair right here that I can hold on to all right are we ready we're going to hinge here we're going to come forward and I'm now we're going to place my hands on the Block and I'm going to let my head fall just a little bit further okay now from this position let's turn the block to the number two position and see

if we can let our heart fall any further oh yeah can we move it to the number one position oh my goodness right now if it feels okay for you you're going to let go of the block and you're going to grab your elbows and you're going to hang out in ragdoll not your head yes shake your head no nod your head yes drop your hands back to the block bend the knees generously and roll it up into standing hold that chair you might be a little a little light-headed my head was down below our heart right that might

have given us a little light-headedness so you don't ever have to do that you can always leave the head above the heart okay we're going to do that one more time this time when we get down into our rag doll I encourage you to bend your knees pretty generously and let's see if we can move the stretch from our legs into our back let's do it let's go ahead and start though with that block on the end that number three position or you're using the chair or you're using your legs right as you go down you can just grab your legs if you don't have the block okay are we ready here we go this is it this is the last thing hinge belly tight you can place your hands in the seat of the chair if you wish you can place your hands on the Block if you wish okay so we're going to hang out here first right we're just hanging out here and breathing feeling the stretch in the back side of the body let's go ahead and move down into that number two position for that block or your hands are going down on your legs a little further all right are we ready we're going to go to that number one position if it's okay to let your head fall do so I'm kind of looking at the camera just so I can engage with you guys but if you'll look down and let your head fall that's ideal if it feels okay all right here we go we're going to bend those knees pretty generously you see what I'm doing there I'm bending those knees pretty generously my heart Falls a little bit further I'm going to grab my elbows and I'm going to

hang out in ragdoll so the idea here is to try to get the stretch out of the legs and into the back okay do you feel that not your head yes shake your head no not the head yes drop the hands to the to the block or the chair or whatever now we're going to roll it up keep those knees bent and we're going to roll it up into standing hold that chair very good let's come to seated oh man I felt that felt let's see all step um move your hips all the way back hands are resting lightly on the thighs Palms are facing up take a deep breath

in and a full breath out close your eyes shavasana pose let life be let the little things bring you Joy let the big things give you inspiration let the challenges make you more determined let the problems bring out your skills let your differences with others build a pathway to new understanding let your fears show you how to exercise your courage let the noise and confusion teach you to be more focused let the annoyances distractions and interruptions strengthen your patience let the new moments come

let the past go let experience show up and teach you its lessons let life be as life will be and let yourself grow more alive more capable more purposeful and effective as a result take a deep breath in and a full breath out drop your right ear towards your right shoulder reach up with the right hand give the head a gentle tug as you press that left hand down towards the floor release it drop your chin towards your chest reach up with your hands give the head a gentle tug

release it drop your left ear towards your left shoulder reach up with the left hand give the head a gentle tug pressing that right hand down towards the floor release it look out just slightly open your mouth if you want to stretch your jaw bring your hands to your heart

DAY 15

let's get started so we're going to sit up nice and tall in our chair maybe you move forward a little bit definitely don't be leaning back let's take a moment now to focus on that mind and body and breath we're going to ground our feet to the Earth thinking about having both feet on the floor equally weighted and the same thing with our sits Minds right so we have those six months equally weighted on the chair let's take our hands place them lightly on the thighs flip those Palms up to the ceiling lift your heart lower your shoulders close your eyes or soften the eyes and just breathe so we take a few moments here at the

beginning of our practice to connect to that breath feeling your natural inhalation and exhalation let's begin to elongate the breath inhaling a little more deeply exhaling a little more completely do that again inhale and exhale now we're going to move that breath down into our diaphragm as we inhale the belly extends we're filling those lungs from the bottom up and as we exhale actively pull the belly button in towards the spine pushing the air up and out of the lungs do that a couple more times and breathe normally

bring your hands to your heart set your intentions for today's practice one more breath here bring your hands back down to your thighs and open your eyes very very okay we're gonna look to the right just a little neck stretch here and then we're going to like Center and we're going to look to the left and let's center now we're going to do that again so we're going to look back to the right and then just take that gaze a little further over those shoulders not the head just the Gaze

just the the eyes right and look Center and let's go the other side so again get your head as far around as feels comfortable for you and then just take your gaze a little further over that shoulder and release that let's bring our hands down by our side and shrug those shoulders up into the ears and then we're just going to let them fall so that a little bit of gravity helping us there here we go shrug up and down let's do that one more time shrug it up and just let them fall that feels good all right so now I'm

gonna do just a little neck stretch here so we're going to let that ear fall towards the shoulder so just feel your natural range of motion here for that next stretch now we're going to reach up with that hand and you're just going to lay it lightly on the head don't pull or tug then take the opposite arm extend it out flexing through the wrist pushing through the heel of the hand oh that feels good one more breath here let's bring the hand down take the hand off of the head and then bring that head

up take a moment ha right okay we're going to the other side so we're going to let that left ear fall down towards that left shoulder so just hang out here for a few breaths feeling that natural stretch your range of motion here now we're going to lift up with that hand and we're just going to lay it lightly on the head so again don't pull or tug it's just the weight of the hand that's going to give that head just a little more stretch and then the final piece is adding that extended arm so it's out to the side

Flex through the wrist push through the heel of the hand and feel that stretch oh boy all right let's bring that hand down take the hand off of the head lift that head up do you want to do another shoulder shrug I do and let's release it one more time shrug it up and release so we're going to do an extended Mountain variation we're going to extend our arms out to the side okay so it's kind of like we call these uh Warrior two arms so remember shoulders are down a little activeness in those arms so squeeze the

muscles against the bones so acting like you're going to hold me up if I tried to pull your arms down right you feel that okay now we're going to flip those Palms up to the ceiling little different stretch shoulders stay down belly is tight flipping back down towards the floor take the arms up to the ceiling now we're going to take my right arm to the chair and I'm going to extend my left arm up now I'm going to lean over my mountain now take your hand and flip it up towards the ceiling turn and look up

now let's learn that mountain again hand is on the chair for support take that right arm up I'm sorry left arm up and let's do that one more time arm up we go and release okay we're gonna do that whole series again for the other side here we go extended Mountain variation we're going to extend our arms wide like Warrior two arms remember they're active I'm pulling my muscles in against the bones I'm activating the upper body here shoulders are down belly is tight flip the Palms up towards the ceiling

we got it back down towards the floor arms up to the ceiling now we're going to do the other side here we go hand down to the chair extend that opposite arm and let's lean so this feeling you should have a stretch from the hip tip to the armpit and the armpit all the way out that hand so it's two very distinct feeling stretches do you feel that all right now we're going to take this hand and we're going to take it up to the ceiling turn and look up all right let's do that again lean hand to the ceiling turn and look up

we're gonna do that one more time lean you've got your opposite hand on that chair to give you some support so you can lean a little deeper into it turn and look up bring that hand down and release very good so the next pose is body Circle so I'm going to have my hands on my thighs to give me some support and I'm going to lean forward all right so you might feel a little stretch in the back here all right now let's go to the side and now we're going to come back so as you come back don't rest on the

back of the chair make your abdominals do some work here and then we're going to come over to the side and we're going to come forward and we're going to do that again just like that to the side back side and forward and now we're going to reverse our Circle okay so now we're going to go the other way don't skimp on this back part right make your abdominals work to the side there's the obliques working and Center let's do that again oh yeah I feel it do you okay now let's come up and we're going

to just do that one more time in each direction we're going to add a little breath in there and remember if at any time you don't want to add the the you know the yoga breath and you're just going to breathe normally just don't hold your breath okay here we go inhale as we come forward exhale to the side inhale back exhale to the side let's do that again inhale exhale inhale and exhale reverse it here we go inhale and exhale just take your time here feeling all of those muscles working right feeling everything in those side

waist muscles now those abdominals are working and adding that breath in and release all right excellent work so the next pose and next series we've done the sun salutation now quite a bit so what we're adding today is chair pose now in our chair pose we're going to start pretty simply by like acting like we're going to get up out of the chair but not then we'll get all the way up out of the chair so just take your time we're going to build and remember you don't ever have to add on

right so you can keep doing the same version you don't have to add the the additional piece on and I'll cue those add-ons and you can always do the previous version okay so I don't know if you've noticed but I just brought my feet back just a little bit so here's the thing if you've got your feet way back out here and you have your hands at heart and you try to get up out of the tube right it's very very difficult if even possible so what I want you to think about is bringing your feet back now you always

want the knees behind the toes right so you want to be able to see those toes but now you can press so what you want to be able to do is press down as you lift okay so let's go ahead and get those feet in the right position we'll bring our hands to heart now we're going to inhale as we come up to our Mountain pose and then we're going to bring our hands back to heart on an exhale inhale we're going to come up exhale we're going to dive forward forward salute airplane arms we've done this when we

know it well inhale we're going to bring hands to the thighs and let that heart fall forward tuck the chin roll it up we're going to do that one more time bring hands to Heart ready big circle up we go bring your hands to heart back up to Mountain pose dive forward forward salute airplane arms let's stretch that out and let's do that supported forward fold tuck that chin roll it up and bring your hands to your heart we're going to add in as chair pose but we're not going to get up out of the chair we're going to

act like we are but we're not going to ready here we go big circle up we go Mountain pose bring your hands to Heart let's come back up dive it forward forward salute our plane arms we're going to stretch let's come to that forward fold all right are we ready bring your hands to your heart inhale to prepare exhale act like you're getting out of the chair but don't so my quadriceps are very engaged my abdominals are very engaged my shoulders are down out of my ears my hands are at heart one more breath

release let's do that again big circle up Mountain pose bring your hands to Heart let's come back to Mountain pose come into that forward salute airplane arms we've got this forward fold let's let that heart fall forward are we ready for that chair pose again hands to Heart inhale to prepare act like you're going to get out of the chair but don't take one more breath and release okay how does that feel all right so we're going to do that again and this time we're actually going

to get up out of the chair let's all give that a try before we do the whole series so bring your hands to Heart pull your belly in now an option here is to have your hands on your thighs right so you can inhale to prepare exhale you can push up with your hands on thighs and then bring your hands to heart that's a great option okay or go ahead and sit back down you can have hands at heart inhale to prepare exhale come up into your chair pose and let's come back down to see it okay so I'm gonna let you pick which version

of that you like to do I'll do one each way listen we're going to go through this two more times before we add more on you're like oh my gosh all right are we ready big circle up we go to Mountain pose bring your hands to Heart let's come back to Mountain pose and we're going to dive forward forward salute airplane arms stretch hands on those thighs for that supported forward fold okay are we ready now in how to prepare Place those hands on those thighs come into your chair pose bring your hands to Heart okay so a

couple of things now what I want you to be looking thinking about is your knees are behind your toes and I want you to be able to lift those toes up off the floor and wiggle them okay so the weight is back you see what's happening here my weight is shooting back I'm not bringing my knees forward right I'm bringing my hips back belly is tight at the work is happening in those quadriceps do y'all see that okay let's take a deep breath in and on an exhale we're going to sit back down did you feel that quadriceps

right I know let's do it again big circle up we go let's bring those hands to Heart we're going to come back up into our Mountain pose and we're going to dive forward forward salute airplane arms stretch it let's come to that forward fold let that heart fall forward inhale to prepare bring your hands to Heart take a deep breath in come into your chair pose one more breath here come to standing reverse Swan Dive up we go bring your hands to heart back up we go dive It Forward High forward salute airplane

arms stretch it out ready for that forward fold hands on thighs bend your knees hands back to Heart there we are in our chair pose again right inhale to prepare exhale sit back down let's do that one more time just like that up we go bring your hands to Heart we're going to come back up to Mountain posing we're going to dive it forward forward salute airplane arms let's go into that forward fold are we ready take a deep breath in on an exhale press up into your chair pose hello feeling it I am one more breath stand up reverse

one type all the way to Mountain pose bring your hands to Heart come back up to Mountain pose dive it forward forward salute airplane arms stretch forward fold hands to Heart Bend those knees into that chair pose that was my knee that just cracked I don't know if you heard that I did one more breath have a seat and turn please how did you do did you feel pretty good on that one I know it's challenging right adding that chair pose is challenging okay we're going to come to standing uh I'm gonna do it beside my chair I don't

know I think beside the chair is going to be better if you feel like you're a little more stable Behind the Chair that's always an option but I'm going to do mine beside the chair so this is going to be Eagle legs to Warrior three pose now I'm going to hold my chair here and I'm going to put my weight into the leg that's next to the chair okay now the other leg I'm going to create a table top so my knee is lifted my foot is flexed I'm going to refer to this as an eagle leg just to help us with what what we're

doing here with this series so I'm going to refer to this as eagle leg so when I say come to eagle leg it's basically lifting the knee up into tabletop does that make sense okay so now let's try this one before we let go of the chair okay so what I want you to do is I want you to take this foot that's in the air and I want to push it through back behind you to Warrior three now notice let's bring one hand to heart so we're going to come to prayer hands here in a minute but let's hold the chair to begin with so what I

want you to think about is I'm not I'm not down here right my heart is lifted and I'm making my glute and my hamstring do the work here there's a lot of work happening in that leg and then we're going to bring that knee back up okay let's do that one more time just like that holding on to that chair push that foot through hanging out here come back up and put that foot down Okay so let's take a moment here we're going to do that same Series without holding on to the chair so a little bit of balance work but the good

thing is as you've got the chair here right so maybe you let go and you hold it and you let go and you hold it so that's a way for you to begin to build into that balance practice okay so here we go let's bring that knee up we've got that foot flexed our belly is tight so one of the key things for balance is abdominals keeping your belly tight lifting up through those pelvic floor muscles are we ready we're going to let go of the chair we're going to bring hands to Heart hello just hanging out here we're breathing

hanging out and breathing okay are we ready we're gonna push that leg through to that Warrior three now that's a dynamic balance move anytime we move in Balance it's very challenging right it's easier sometimes I think to just stand stay put they're just different one static and one's Dynamic let's bring that knee back up and we're gonna put that foot down mindfully so let's move to the other side of the chair while I chat for a second so anytime we get out of a pose we want to make sure if we're getting

out of a balance post that it's on purpose with intention right so if you fall out of it and don't get back into it on purpose then you haven't really made any progress in that balance series okay and that ability to hold those Balance poses so we want to make sure that we get out of it mindfully okay so let's come back up we're going to bring that knee up calling this that eagle leg let's go ahead and push it through before we let go of the chair if you want to bring one hand to heart because that's where

it's going to be when we release the chair let's bring that knee up so a little bit of dynamic movement so here we're static and then we push through into that Dynamic so it's very challenging to move all right are we ready bring that knee up or let's let go of that chair if we feel like it's okay hands to Heart belly tight right okay are we ready we're going to inhale if you want to add that breath exhale as we push that leg through then we're going to come up and then we're going to push that foot

through and we're going to do that one more time up we go and we're going to push that foot through then we're going to bring the knee up and we're going to put the foot down mindfully okay very good so let's come back to the other side we're just going to add one more thing to this and so we've had our hands at heart and we've moved our leg now we're going to move our arms I know it's challenging but let's get into it okay so let's bring that knee up I'm holding my chair

belly is tight okay are we ready we're gonna let go of that chair now we're going to push that foot through into that Warrior three and then we're going to bring those Arms by our side airplane arms hello one more breath here come back up and put that foot down let's do that one more time are we ready knee comes up hands to Heart push the foot through bring those Arms by your side airplane arms for three and two and one bring that knee up and put that foot down let's do the other side good balance work here okay are we ready

bring that knee up bring your hands to Heart belly tight are we ready push that foot through let's bring that knee up let's do that again push the foot through to that Warrior three okay we're gonna add on bring the knee up now we're going to add those Eagle arms or airplane arms here we go push it through add the airplane arms heart is lifted bring the knee up and let's do that again push through into those

Eagle uh airplane arms why do I keep saying Eagle airplane arms up we go one more time here we go press it

through airplane arms heart is lifted three three two one up we go and release very good okay come to the other side of your chair we're going to do a sun salutation B which is adding in our chair pose all right so hands to Heart we're going to reverse Swan Dive all the way up and we're going to bring our hands to Heart remember that's the exhale if you want to add the breath inhale up we go exhale forward salute airplane arms stretch let's put our hands on our thighs for a supported forward fold

now bend your knees push your hips back bring your hands to heart into chair pose all right remember hips are back right knees are behind toes I can wiggle my toes my heart is lifted often I'll see in my classes my in-person classes people will be here I really want you to lift up it makes you work your abdominals and your quads more when you have when you lift that heart up do you feel that all right are we ready we're going to stand come up to Mountain pose dive forward hi halfway lift inhale exhale support it forward fold high and

then we're going to bend those knees and come into that chair pose now this time we're going to forward fold now if it feels okay instead of holding your thighs you're going to go ahead and forward forward fold hands towards the floor now we're going to reverse one die bring your arms out and around Palms are facing up as we lift up into Mountain pose if that's too much on your back you're just going to roll up it's okay bring your hands to heart you don't have to do that arms extended out you can

just roll up slowly back up we go to Mountain pose belly button to spine and we're going to dive forward again Swan Dive let's place our hands on our thighs and do a halfway lift extending through the spine nice and long and now we're going to do that forward fold all the way down if that feels okay now bend your knees hands to Heart chair pose how's that feel very tight one more breath let's go ahead and forward fall one more time I know and let's reverse one dive up so my arms are out to the side Palms face up

towards the ceiling and we're going to bring our hands to our excellent work okay let's come to seated all right let's take our right leg extended out long toes to the ceiling we're going to lengthen through our spine and let our heart fall forward so there's pyramid pose that should feel pretty good we work those hamstrings a bit didn't we and Tuck that chin and roll it up and let's do that again nice long spine let that heart fall forward and we're going to tuck the chin and

roll it up and let's just go to the other side opposite leg extends toes to the ceiling lengthen through the spine holding on to those thighs let that heart fall forward tuck that chin and roll it up and we're going to do that one more time nice long spine heart Falls forward back is flat I'm looking out not down one more breath and up we go very very good work okay let's sit back in our chair moving into shavasana pose hands are resting lightly on the thighs Palms are flipped up to there's a

ceiling I'm going to close my eyes and I'm going to take a deep breath in and a full breath out this is when whatever else you have or do not have you have now you have the experience of this moment Perhaps it is painful or maybe it is comfortable most likely it's somewhere in between yet no matter the nature of this moment of this experience it has value now and and only now is your chance to live that value step away from any thoughts or feelings that push you out of the moment see right now for the opportunity it is

for the depth of life it contains this is when you can understand this is when you can experience this is when you can act this is when you can live the past is gone future is a mere concept and all that is everything you are is right now be fully in the best way you can imagine take a deep breath in and a full breath out drop your right ear towards your right shoulder reach up with the right hand give the head a gentle tug pressing that left hand down towards the floor release it

drop your chin towards your chest reach up with your hands give the head a gentle tug release it drop your left ear towards your left shoulder reach up with the left hand give the head a gentle tug pressing that right hand down towards the floor release it look up just slightly open your mouth if you want to stretch your jaw bring your hands to your heart honoring one another we say namaste thank you so much for joining today my fellow bottoms downies we've made it to the end of day 15. don't you agree the hardest part is just getting to your chair once we're here isn't it just wonderful please keep showing up

DAY 16

let's get started so we're going to sit up nice and tall in our chair we're moving forward we're not leaning back we're going to take our feet and ground them to the Earth this is our time that we connect that mind and body and Breath Right ground those sits bones onto the chair make sure they're equally weighted lift your heart lower your shoulders out of your ears place your hands lightly on the thighs flip the Palms up to the ceiling close your eyes and just breathe so just connecting to that breath and with each inhalation I want you to think about making the spine a little longer as you inhale think about lengthening

through the spine and maybe a deeper breath and breathe normally bring your hands to your heart set your intentions for today's practice bring your hands down to your thighs open your eyes and moving on we're going to take our shoulders and we're going to shrug them up into our ears and then we're going to bring them back and then we're going to bring them down and then we're going to do that again we're going to shrug up into the ears and bring them back and down one more time shrug up

bring them back and down all right very very good I just like I'm just going to move my head a little side to side just a little next stretch there it feels good to me all right so let's go ahead and just let our left ear fall towards our left shoulder and just can't kind of hang out here for a moment and feel that stretch and then we're going to bring the head up and then we're just going to do the other side just a little stretch there for that neck now let's look up just slightly a little

bit of openness through the throat look forward and then let's just let that head fall for a moment and release okay excellent so we're going to move into a goddess pose series and add in some shoulder dip so we'll do a heel and a toe heel toe so you want those feet to be pretty wide all right so at least the width of the chair legs I prefer if you can get a little bit wider and feel comfortable but let's make sure we don't let the knees fold in so if you need to bring the feet in a little bit more to keep the knees in

alignment I would prefer you to have the feet in and keep those knees in alignment okay does that make sense good deal so we're going to take our right shoulder first we're going to hold on to those thighs and we're going to let that right shoulder just dip down between our legs should feel pretty good okay then we're going to come up and now we're going to do the other side so we're just going to let that left shoulder it just kind of dips down between those knees see how when I'm

kind of it's a little bit of a Twist if you will just a gentle one here though and then up we go okay let's do that again one more time just like that to get a feel of it before we add on so I'm going to let that shoulder dip down I don't know about you but I'm feeling a little sideways my abdominals are tight here feeling a little stretched through the shoulder up we go and let's do the other side and up we go okay so the add-on here I'm going to go ahead and drop my shoulder down now I want you to take this hand so

this is my right shoulder is dropping down take your right hand I want you to push on the inside of that right knee so I'm pushing my knee open wider I'm feeling a little more of a stretch in the groin I've got to stretch in the side waist and the shoulder I don't know what you're feeling but that's what I'm particularly feeling and it feels good and let's come up ha ready for the other side let's drop that shoulder down and let's push just getting a little extra stretch in

there our breath and up we go let's do that one more time ha just feels good and up we go last one shoulder dips push against that inner thigh feel that stretch and release let's he'll tell those feet back in together how's that feel a little stretch there for the groin and the side waist it feels good to me so we're going to move into an extended Mountain pose and then from that mountain pose we're going to come into staff pose so let's extend our Mountain first shoulders your down belly is tight

fingertips to the ceiling right we've done this when we know this one well okay so now what I want you to do is you're going to bring your thumbs right under the arms and I want you to lift up this is a pose that looks pretty simple but when you feel it and do it with with uh intention really it really has an impact so I'm lifting up right belly is tight now I want you to maintain this extended this lift let go and bring your hands to the chair staff pose one more breath and release did you feel

that how that lifts okay let's do it again we're going to come up to Extended Mountain lengthen nice and long shoulders are down out of the ears all right are we ready bring your hands right under the arms lift up and release hands to the chair don't release the extension just release the hands from under the arms one more breath and release last time let's do it extend shoulders are down hands under the arms lift up belly tight ready we're going to release under the hands under the arms place them on the

chair staff pose and release again you watch somebody do that and you're thinking yeah whatever until you do it and then you really feel what's happening there so the next series is something that's going to really focus in on those abdominals okay so I have moved forward in my chair quite a bit okay now I want you to lean all the way back so I'm resting on the back of my chair and I'm going to cross my arms at chest your feet are staying on the floor knees are bent inhale to prepare exhale you're

going to lift up do not let those feet come up off the floor inhale we're going to come back now we're not going to rest we're going to touch the back of that chair but we're not resting and then exhale we're going to come up and let's do that again back we go and up we go and back are you feeling your abdominals working here and up two more backrest do not rest I'm sorry touch do not rest enough last one we got this and release okay so that's a great diversion and if you want to stick with

that version go for it if you want a little add-on with me we're going to bring our hands back behind our head elbows are back okay so the elbows aren't coming forward they're staying back and I'm not pulling on my head is just resting lightly in the palms of my hands all right are we ready inhale back we go touch the chair don't rest exhale up we go do you feel the difference right inhale back keeping those feet down exhale up inhale back exhale up we got a few more back we go up we go back

and up can we do one more back and all right you feel that so now we're going to do just a little bit for those oblique muscles so I'm going to take my right leg and I'm going to extend it long bring your hands to your heart and you're going to twist and maybe that left elbow comes down towards the seat of the chair it doesn't have to touch and then you're going to come up and bring that knee in and then we're going to go to the other side extending the leg twisting elbow towards the seat of the chair and up we

go let's do the other side twist and up other side twist and up again twist and up last one last side we've got this twist and up and release so a little oblique work there did you feel that yeah right okay so we're gonna do a crescent lunge today which we've done before but we're gonna do a little add-on to our Crescent lunch so we're going to take this right knee and open it we've done this one we know it right left knee is going to fall down towards the floor we know this one too push that foot back

okay so we're gonna bring our hands to our heart take your hands up to the ceiling now starting with your left arm you're going to Windmill around to face me you're going to take the hands up to the ceiling and then you're going to Windmill them around to face the back of your chair and then you're going to take the hands to the ceiling you're going to come to goal post arms squeeze your shoulder blades back behind you looking up slightly fingertips back to the ceiling bring the hands back down to the chair

and release okay now let's do the other side like that before we add on so let's go ahead and we're going to take the left knee and open it right knee falls down towards the floor push the foot back bring your hands to Heart so remember I'm up on those back toes I'm feeling a pretty good stretch on the front side of that back leg okay are we ready hands to the ceiling here we go we're going to Windmill to face me and hands to the ceiling Windmill and face the other way and hands to the ceiling

goal post arms squeeze your shoulder blades behind you look up hands to the ceiling bring the hands down and release okay very very good so now the little bit of that well it's not a little left out it's quite a big animal but let's do it so we're going to take this right knee and open it we're going to let that left knee fall down towards the floor now here's what we're going to do we're going to scoot out just a little bit hold that chair and let your hips come off of the chair oh yeah there we are

you feel that so hold that chair for right now get your balance remember belly tight abdominals are going to help your balance lifting up through those pelvic floor muscles okay are we ready we're going to bring our hands to Heart exhale as you bring your hands to the ceiling inhale to prepare exhale you're going to turn and face me hello hands to the ceiling now you're going to turn and face over your chair hands to the ceiling go post arms squeeze your shoulder blades behind you look up belly tight hands back to the

ceiling bring your hand to the chair slip your hips back on and face forward how'd you do on that one I know it's challenging I'm giving you some challenge today okay let's do the other side so we're going to open that left knee first right let the right knee fall down screwed out now if you feel like you want to give it a try you're going to slip your hips off of that chair we're going to pull that belly in we're going to bring our hands to Heart bend that front knee right okay extend those arms up now we're

going to Windmill and face me hands to the ceiling Windmill and face over your chair hands to the ceiling go post arms squeeze those shoulder blades behind looking up one more breath and release slip your hips back on that chair and face forward take a moment here you feeling okay I know that one was challenging okay we're going to come to standing on the right side of our chair now again you're going to be standing on the right side of the chair and you're we're going to first come into a mountain pose and then we're

going to lean our mountain and we're going to do a little balance by lifting our leg off the floor as we lean okay so let's start by just bringing our hands to heart you're going to want to have those feet a good solid hit distance apart all right so you want some space between those feet let's bring our hands to our heart okay now we're going to come up into extended Mountain Palms are together interlace your fingers pointer finger is up to the ceiling now we're going to lean our Mountain towards our chair

and then we're going to come up and we're going to lean our Mountain away from our chair and we're going to come up and we're going to lean our Mountain one more time towards our chair and then this time if you want we're going to lift that right leg up off the floor just a little bit right maybe the toes stay down maybe the toes don't one more breath here we're going to come back up to standing and we're going to bring our hands down okay let's do the other side so we're going to start

with the weight with our feet about hip distance apart right and we're going to bring our hands to Heart we're going to come all the way up to that ex Mountain pose extended Mountain interlace fingers pointer finger to the ceiling we're going to lean in towards our chair and then we're going to come up and we're going to lean away from our chair now we're going to come up let's lean towards our chair again and up lean away from the chair I know we're about to add that leg lift are we

ready okay here we go let's lean towards our chair now you're going to lift this leg up remember you can have toes on the floor if that feels better for you or you can lift that foot up for a little extra balance work belly tight one more breath bring the foot in bring the hands up and arms come down all right very good did that feel okay it's a little work on that balance right a little standing balance pose there okay so we're going to move into a downward facing dog we'll start with our downward

facing puppy now here's the thing it's really important that your chair is on carpet or maybe it's on us like a yoga mat like a sticky mat what I want you to think about is pressing down on that chair not out so I don't want the chair to slide out from under you okay so first is better the best thing is it's being a carpet or a sticky mat the second best is making sure you're pressing down and not out okay so we want to do that anyway we want to press down not out anyway okay so I'm going to take a step away from my

chair so it's not a huge step just a little step away now I'm going to begin hinging right at the hips right and then I'm going to bring my hands into the seat of the chair and I'm going to bring my weight forward okay so we're going to start with a downward puppy and so what I'm going to do now is instead of my hands being on my Palms I'm going to bring them down onto my forearms are you feeling your back stretching already let's go ahead and take another step back not a big one another step back

remember you're pressing down not out then I want you to push your hips back behind you my heart Falls I'm looking down if that feels okay on your neck right so we're not keeping the head up we're letting the head come down you should be feeling a quite a stretch through the back side of the body my hips are high my heart is falling I'm going to take three more breaths here another breath here and last breath okay so as we come out of it I want you to bend your knees step forward then hold that chair and roll up okay so

how did that feel now if you want to stick with downward facing puppy if you like it better on your forearms that's absolutely fine if you want to try it on your palms that's another version right so and then and both of them are great so let's take a step back first okay remember we're hinging at our hips coming forward placing your hands on the seat of the chair bringing the weight forward so my shoulders are over my wrist and then if you're coming down your shoulders are still over your

elbows here okay so the weight comes forward all right are we ready we're going to lift our hips High we're going to push our heart back I'm going to take one more step back just for me if you don't want to take a step back it's okay but what I'm going to let my heart fall forward oh yeah and I'm feeling that pretty significant stretch in the back side of the body my belly is tight I have one more breath here and I'm going to bring my weight forward and I'm going to step forward step forward and

roll it up okay now we're going to add two things on and remember you don't ever have to add on but the first thing we're going to do if you want to peek at me real quick we're going to be in our down dog right so then I'm going to take a hand off the chair and I'm going to bring it to my heart and then I'll put it down and then I'll do the other side then I'm going to take a leg up for a three-legged dog and I'm going to put it down and then I'll do the other side and put it down okay so

don't do them if you don't want to it's okay you can just stick with your down dog or your down puppy if you don't want to add on all right but if you're with me here we go haha I'm gonna hinge forward right and we'll place my hands in that chair and I'm going to step back I'm gonna let my heart fall forward my hips go high sinking down into your downward facing dog or puppy okay so here I am in my down dog my heart is lower is is kind of between my arms my I'm feeling that stretch I'm going to

release the chair from with my right hand and I'm going to touch my heart it doesn't matter which one you do first we're going to do both then we're going to bring that hand back to the chair we're going to release and touch the other hand the other hand to the heart and release okay we ready for three-legged dog here we go one leg lifts up for three-legged dog belly tight one more breath bring that foot back to the floor lift the other foot up for that three-legged dog bringing that foot down step forward

and roll up into a standing position all right how did that feel that feel pretty good I down dog I think that's a good one maybe not all the add-ons right you're like we could have just stuck a down dog but okay so now the next thing we're going to do again that chair is on that carpet or on that sticky mat or make sure you're pressing down not out we're going to take our leg next to the back of the chair and I'm going to bring that foot up into the chair so hold on okay now I'm gonna you know I'm gonna take

this step I'm gonna take a step back with this leg so I'm going to bring my foot back down I'm going to take a step back and then I'm ready and I'll tell you why I did that but I want this knee to stay behind those toes and so I just kind of needed I needed that uh this foot to be back just a little bit so kind of see what works for you take a moment here I want you to have this foot in the chair but we're going to push forward and as we push our hips forward I want to make sure this knee stays

behind those toes okay so kind of find what works for you okay are we ready so we're going to start in pyramid pose though so we're going to straighten the front leg first holding that chair toes come up and I'm going to hinge forward so there's my pyramid pose so there's the back side of that leg right you feel that we're hanging out here we've got a straight leg so don't bend the knee we tend to every you know I know people want to bend the knee so they can get that heart lower I'd rather you keep the

legs straight it doesn't matter how far the heart comes down but the minute you bend the knee you've disengage it's part of that hamstring and so we want that whole muscle set to stretch okay now let's come forward I'm going to push my hips forward and there's a version of Crescent lunge do you feel that stretch here I know me too oh my goodness right ah okay let's do that again pyramid pose Toast of the ceiling let that heart fall forward feeling that stretch in the back of that leg

okay let's come forward pyramid I mean uh Crescent lunge oh man that feels good pushing those hips forward getting that stretch right here my heart is lifted I'm breathing I'm not holding my breath and release excellent work okay let's go to the other side so now I'm going to do this first I'm going to take that little step back and then I'm going to bring that foot up just you know you know where we're headed with this now so make sure that knee's going to be behind those toes when you push forward okay so let's

start in pyramid I'm holding my chair I'm going to straighten this front leg my toes are up to the ceiling hold on let that heart fall forward so here's the other thing you might find this side more willing than the other or less willing this is my less willing sign okay that's why I mentioned it because I was like oh boy all right so now I'm going to bend that knee and I'm gonna push my hips forward oh yeah so again making sure you're pushing down right so we don't want to be pushing

away with that chair we want that even though my weight coming forward I still want that foot pushing down okay let's come back pyramid pose again and forward Crescent lunge ah one more time pyramid pose inhale to prepare exhale letting that heart fall forward and Crescent one more breath and relax all right let's come back to seated pose well it's not really a poses images coming back to seated hear what I mean not what I say okay so now I'm going to take I'm going to move into pigeon pose so remember you've got options you can leave this left leg right where it is and you can cross your right ankle over to that other ankle right so you you're ankle to ankle or if it feels okay you can do ankle to knee so just feel what feels good for for you what works for you but this is the area of the body we should be feeling stretching back into that hip and glute area let's extend nice and long through the spine begin to let that heart fall forward go ahead and tuck your chin roll it up and then I want you to just move this

knee a little bit up and down so really it's for the hip so right we're moving that hip joint a little okay let's extend through the spine inhale to prepare exhale you're going to let the heart fall forward and maybe you press gently on that leg you don't have to it's just an option and up we go and let's move that leg up and down a little last time let's do it come forward now another option you can do is bring your arms out first and then let them fall down towards the floor

that's another good stretch if that feels good do this one if this one feels better doesn't matter they're all really good okay we got to do the other side so remember if you want to do that ankle to ankle then that's a great version you just stay right here you'll still do all the you know the lip the heart forward but if you want to do ankle to knee then that's another option okay so we're hanging out here for just a moment let's just kind of get them let the body settle into the pose and then

when we're ready extend the spine nice and long and begin to let that heart fall forward and then we're going to tuck that chin and roll it up and then we're going to do that again nice long spine if you want to press gently on that leg you can hold that hold the movement not the breath right we're breathing just a natural inhale and exhale here feel that stretch and up we go let's move that knee a little bit up and down and then the final version if you like it you can come actually up and out

and then hands down just one more breath here all right let's all come back up to seated put your feet on the floor go ahead and lean back moving into shavasana pose hands resting lightly on the thighs flip the Palms up to the ceiling inhale to prepare and as you exhale close your eyes and feel yourself just melting into the chair early start early morning holds the power of the whole day ahead welcome that power embody it make use of it a good night's rest has refreshed your senses and transformed yesterday's challenges into today's strength early morning introduces that new Strength to the new day of opportunities start early with the day invigorated by the prospect of working through New Challenges as the day brightens feel your Effectiveness grow while the day's possibilities still seem endless sees firmly upon some of them this isn't an ideal time to do what matters to do what satisfies your desires to make a difference join in eagerly as the world comes to life celebrate and appreciate all over again

the wonder that stretches out in every direction give yourself the advantage of an early start tap into the early morning magic that dances before your eyes take a deep breath in and a full breath out drop your right ear towards your right shoulder reach up with the right hand give the head a gentle tug as you press that left hand down towards the floor release it drop your chin towards your chest reach up with the hands give the head a gentle tug release it drop your left ear towards your left

shoulder reach up with the left hand give the head a gentle tug pressing the right hand down towards the floor release it look out just slightly open your mouth if you want to stretch your jaw bring your hands to your heart

DAY 17

let's get started so we're going to start by sitting up nice and tall in our chair we're going to move forward not leaning back take a moment focusing in on that mind and body and breath taking our feet grounding them to the Earth right thinking about having both of them equally weighted on the floor also with those sits Bones on the chair nice and grounded equally weighted we're gonna lift our heart up pull the shoulders down out of the ears flip those Palms up to the ceiling close the eyes and breathe so we're connecting to that breath that natural inhalation and exhalation we'll move that breath down into the diaphragm as we inhale the belly extends

we're filling the lungs from the bottom up and as we exhale pulling the belly button in towards the spine pushing the air up and out of the lungs so do that a couple of times and just breathe normally bring your hands to your heart set your intentions for today's practice or breath here bring your hands back down to your thighs and open your eyes and we're going to roll those shoulders forward up back and down let's do that again forward up back and down and then reverse it ah yeah you got it one more time

we're going to let our ear fall towards our shoulder now I want you to grab the back of the chair and squeeze your shoulder blades behind you oh yeah you feel that a little different way to stretch into the neck and let's release that ha let's do the other side so we let our ear fall to the shoulder they're going to reach back grab the chair squeeze the shoulder blades back behind you feel that stretch okay let's release that now one final thing we're going to do chin to chest we're going to reach back

grab the chair squeeze the shoulder blades behind you and release all right let's do a heel toe heel toe so we've got those feet nice and wide and we're just going to do some simple shoulder dips so we're going to drop that shoulder down between the legs so there's a nice stretch sideways I'll fill it a little into my back and up in the shoulder and then we're going to come up hands are going to rest here on those thighs for some support and then we're going to let that other

shoulder dip down and up we go let's do that again down lift the shoulder up and let's do that again just dropping that shoulder down between the legs and up and then one more time oh yeah should feel good lifting up and do that on the other side and if we go very good okay let's he'll tell those feet back together now I'm going to continue with my hands on thighs for support and I'm going to lean forward all right now we're going to go to the side and we're going to circle back and then we're going to go to the other

side and then come forward and let's do that again to the side back other side and forward and now we're going to reverse that so we're going to go the other side other way and back side forward and one more time oh yeah and release all right nice so the Pelt the next thing we're going to do our pelvic tilt and so what I want you to do is reach down and feel these pointy bones right here at the tip of the pelvis you feel those two I call that the pelvic tips the tips of the hip bones okay so I want you to take those and I want you to rock them towards your shoulders so see how I'm kind of rotating there's getting a little tilt in right the hips are going forward now I'm going to take come up to normal long spine and then I'm going to take those and I'm going to rock them towards my knees so now my hips are kind of shooting back and then come back let's do that again tilting and Center and tilt forward and Center one more tilting back and Center and forward and Center all right very very good

we're going to move into yesterday we did good mornings and then we're going to do those again today with another add-on a couple of different add-ons okay so we're going to start moving very forward in our chair let's go ahead and lean all the way back and we're going to rest here for just a moment and we're going to cross our uh arms are at right at the chest Crossing at the chest okay so inhale here to prepare exhale we're going to come up into seated now my feet stay down down and I'm making my abdominals do the

work okay inhale let's come back exhale come up now let's come back as you come back you're touching the chair but not resting and then up and let's do that again down and down and we got one more like this down and now we're going to bring our hands back behind our head elbows are wide inhale back we go and exhale up so keep those knees bent feet on the floor right as we come back we're touching the chair we're not resting and up we go keep the elbows back inhale back we go and exhale up oh yeah I'm not pulling on

my head make the ABS do all the work right inhale back exhale up let's do one more like that inhale back and exhale up okay so now the next uh atom is we're going to extend our legs long it really changes the Dynamics of it the feet have to stay down Okay so we're going to start if you want to go ahead and do your arms cross let's do it just to feel it let's come back and so you feel the difference right with those legs long let's do one more okay ready here we go hands behind the head elbows wide back we go inhale

exhale up now try to touch the chair but don't rest so we want to go all the way back and then up we go we're going to go all the way back and then up we go let's do that one more time all the way back and up we go okay now we're going to bend those knees and if you remember yesterday what we did let's do it let's go ahead and do that one we extended one leg out and then we twisted and tried to touch the elbow to the chair remember that and then we came up and then we did the other side so that's

fine stick with that version if you want now if you want a little bit more what we're going to do is instead of the leg coming to the floor we're going to bring it out and twist and in and Center okay let's switch sides extend out twist come back Center foot down extend out twisting coming up putting the foot down other side extend twist and re-release that all right that was very very good moving on let's come to standing on the right side of our chair and we're going to face the seat of our

chair now the leg is next to the back of the chair the leg is next to the back of the chair I want you to take a little step forward so the foot is under the chair and then when you bend your knee it touches okay now with your other leg you're going to take a step back the heel will be on the mat and your foot will be at a 45 degree angle move your hips around to face the chair bend your front knee bring your hands to heart here's a beautiful Warrior one okay let's extend the arms to the ceiling now we're going to start with our

outside arm our right arm and we're going to Windmill around to a Warrior Two facing me so shoulders are down out of the ears heart is lifted arms are parallel to the mat right so arms aren't up or down they were parallel we're going to flip this front Palm up and reverse our Warrior oh yeah feel that stretch now we're going to come back to Warrior Two and then we're going to take this hand and we're going to place it in the chair for that side angle pose then if you want to bring this arm

across you can you don't have to it's just an option and then let's press back into that Warrior Two we're going to flip that Palm up and back and we're going to come back to our Warrior Two squeeze the muscles against the bones and the arms one more breath and let's release okay we are going to be adding something to that series but I want to do that series on each side first and then we're going to add that last little piece so let's come to the other side and remember the foot next to the back

of the chair the leg this is the leg right we're going to take that foot step it under our chair bend the knee so that you can feel the shin touching the chair when you bend the knee okay now take the other leg step back bring that heel down to the floor so that foot is going to be at a bit of an angle bring your hips forward bend the front knee bring your hands to Heart okay Ara so remember be pulling in nice and tight through the belly lengthening nice and long through the tailbone we want to feel the weight back hands to Heart

let's inhale to prepare extend your arms up on an exhale Warrior one okay now starting with the outside arm you're going to Windmill to that Warrior Two facing me so we're going to flip our front Palm up to the ceiling and we're going to reverse our Warrior up and back now we're going to come back to Warrior two and then we're going to take this hand down to the chair as we lift the heart nice and open through the chest bring bicep by ear if you just so desire you don't have to it's just an option

press back up into that Warrior Two we're going to flip our front Palm up and Back Again and then back to Warrior Two release okay very good so come back to the other side and I want you to peek at me real quick and we're going to add a half moon pose now we'll be in our we'll go through our Warrior one more or two we'll do the whole thing just like normal we'll be here in this Warrior two then what I'm going to do is I'm going to bring my weight over my chair and then I'm going

to lift this opposite leg up so there's our half moon pose okay so we just kind of want you to see where we were headed with that so you're like what is she talking about is challenging it is a balanced pose but the good thing is that we have our chair right so we can kind of hang on to that chair a little bit it's still balanced belly has to stay tight okay let's give it a try and if you don't want to try it leave it out it's an add-on you don't have to do it right okay so I got my foot under the chair I'm

going to bend my front knee back foot steps back right that heel is down bring those hips forward bring the hands to the heart extend those arms for that beautiful Warrior One shoulders are down belly tight extend through that spine right nice long extension through that those hips right so down we pushing those hips down the back of that tailbone down all right ready extend those arms up to the ceiling okay we're going to move to that Warrior Two we're going to flip our front Palm up and back now we're going to come back to our

Warrior Two and we're going to come to that side angle pose so just place that hand in the chair lifting up extending your side angle if you want make sure your chest is open don't let yourself collapse bring that arm back okay we're going to come back to Warrior Two now what I'm going to do is I'm going to push off against this front foot okay pull that belly in push off and then lift your back leg up there we are in a half moon pose we have one more breath now I'm going to bend my front knee put

that back foot back down come back to that Warrior Two and release it okay did that do okay let's do the other side so we're going to place my foot under the chair right not just the foot so when you bend it you touch it take a big step back with that opposite that back leg heel is down hips are forward bend the front knee pull that belly in nice and tight lengthen through that tailbone so don't let that belly just hang here really we're actively pulling it in shoulders are down hands to heart so very active pose so Warriors

are active strength building poses inhale to prepare exhale fingertips to the ceiling and how to prepare exhale move to your Warrior Two facing me looking over those front fingertips we're going to flip that front Palm up and back reversing our Warrior we're going to come back to Warrior two and then that hand is going to come into the chair and we're going to lift up nice and open through that heart let's bring bicep by ear we're going to press back up into our Warrior Two okay are we ready we're gonna inhale to

prepare pull that belly button in push off of this front leg come into that Half Moon in three two one bend the front knee put the back foot back down back into your Warrior Two one more breath here and release I know right it's a challenging pose there's no doubt about it good work so we're going to stay on this side of our chair and we're going to bring our hands back behind us interlace your fingers push your knuckles down towards the floor opening up through the chest all right let's take a deep breath in

here pushing those uh pushing that heart open right let's do that again inhale now as we exhale what we're going to do is we're going to open our arms nice and wide now I'm going to cross one arm on top of the other and I'm going to hug myself then I'm going to bring my elbows up towards the ceiling and then I want to bring them down towards the floor and then I'm going to bring them Center and now I'm going to go back up to the ceiling and I'm just going to open up my arms and I'm going to come up on my

tippy toes my belly is tight a little bit of balance work here one more breath and down we go okay so I want to do that same thing again on this same side all right so let's do it we're going to take our hands and we're going to interlace our fingers and push those hands back behind you I want you to open up through the chest looking up maybe if that feels okay on your neck just an openness for the front side of the body okay now we're going to open our arms now whichever arm we put on top let's do

the other one on top this time hug yourself elbows go up to the ceiling elbows go down towards the floor okay are we ready elbows towards the ceiling we're going to let go bring up fingertips to the ceiling I'm up on my tippy toes my belly is tight my gaze is up one more breath here and down week that was so good you guys excellent work okay let's come back to seated ha right wow okay so we're going to take our right knee and we're going to open it so a little inner thigh stretch here we're going to take that left hand we're

going to open it up nice and wide let's bring it all the way across our body grab the chair lift the crown of the head towards the ceiling then you're going to turn and look over the back of your chair half lord of the fish's pose and let's release that so make sure this knee stays open don't let it fold in okay open it up inhale here exhale come across the body grab the chair inhale as you extend the spine exhale as you twist and look over the back of your chair and then just naturally breathe so we're not

holding the breath we're breathing our natural breath one more and release let's let this knee fall down towards the floor push the foot back lift the heart hold and breathe and release it and we're going to do that one more time back of the kneecap towards the ceiling heart lifts and release let's face forward ah we're gonna do the other side now okay let's do it right excuse me left knee opens up so feel that stretch first a little inner thigh stretch we're going to bring that right arm back

all the way across the body grab the chair crown of the head lips we're going to turn and look over the back of our chair and let's release that and we're going to do that again open we're bringing it across the body grab the chair lift and twist and release we're going to let this knee fall down towards the floor for our Crescent lunge push the foot back you're up on those back toes back of the kneecap towards the ceiling heart is lifted and release and let's do that again and release go ahead and face forward

hi we're going to sit back in our chair and move into our shavasana pose hands are resting lightly on the thighs flip the Palms up to the ceiling take a deep breath in and on an exhalation close your eyes take another deep breath in and full breath out 15 minutes is there something you don't want to do but you know you must can you give it just 15 minutes it's not that much time and it will be over before you know yet in that time you can change your trajectory promise yourself a few minutes then dive into the task

even if you just get a little work done that's the whole lot better than nothing yet there is a good chance you'll do even better than that because once you're making a little progress you might not want to stop whether that ends up being the case or not just give it a shot you might be surprised at what you were able to do give it 15 minutes and you could very well get it done take a deep breath in and a full breath out drop your right ear towards your right shoulder reach up with the right hand

give the head a gentle tug pressing that left hand down towards the floor release it drop the chin towards the chest reach up with your hands give the head a gentle tug release it drop your left ear toward your left shoulder reach up with the left hand give the head a gentle tug pressing that right hand down towards the floor release it look up just slightly open your mouth if you want to stretch your jaw bring your hands to your heart

DAY 18

let's get started so we're going to start sitting up nice and tall and moving forward in our chair so we're not leaning back and we're going to take that moment to focus on the mind and the body and the breath so the first thing we're going to do is ground our feet so thinking about having both of those feet on the floor and equally weighted and the same thing with our six bones so those are on that chair and they're equally weighted and we feel like we're

stable must lift our heart lower the shoulders out of the ears place the hands lightly on your thighs now if you could flip those Palms up to the ceiling see how that feels all right we're going to close our eyes so or you can soften the eyes if you're not keen on totally closing them focusing in on the breath and our heart center let's just feel that natural inhalation and exhalation we're going to move our breath down into the diaphragm as we inhale the belly extends we're filling our lungs from the

bottom up and as we exhale we're going to actively pull the belly button in towards the spine pushing the air up and out of the lungs so do that a few times and breathe normally bring your hands to your heart set your intentions for today's practice one more breath here bring your hands back down to your thighs and open your eyes we're going to look side to side so just taking that gaze over one shoulder and then we're going to come Center and take that gaze over the other shoulder and come Center and let's roll those

shoulders up back and down let's do that again up and reverse it I know so just the other way it doesn't matter right we're just rolling those shoulders feeling that neck stretching a little bit those shoulders stretching just a little bit okay we're going to drop our ear towards our shoulders so I want you to just let this natural range of motion happen here we're just gonna hang out here for a few breaths feeling that stretch on the side of the neck you feel that I do now we're going to drop our chin towards

our chest so we're just looking down at the lap and we're feeling a nice stretch to the back of the neck then we're going to go to the other side so just letting that hang out for a few breaths here one more breath and let's go ahead and lift that head up Wow Let's Roll those shoulders again what do you think maybe one at a time and maybe move that head just a little bit okay very very good let's move into our Mountain pose I know we've done this one a lot just does a good one to warm

up the spine it's just a really good one so we're going to spread those fingers nice and wide our shoulders are down our belly is tight now we're going to come to those GoPro storms and squeeze those shoulder blades back behind you fingertips up to the ceiling we're trying to touch that ceiling one more breathless bring the hands down we're going to do that again just like that here we go spread those fingers ah go post arms squeeze those shoulder blades back behind you feeling that openness through the chest

fingertips to the ceiling remember keeping the shoulders down belly stays tight oh yeah that feels good it's an active movement here right lengthening up pulling the shoulders down and release all right did you feel the stretch happening right it's amazing how much stretch we can get and it doesn't look like we're doing much of anything but we really are okay so now I'm going to take my thumbs to the back wall as I start into my cow pose so think about lifting up just a little bit through the chin

having a nice open throat all right thumbs to that back wall squeezing those shoulder blades behind looking up a little bit if that feels okay and then we're going to round down into our cat pose has on thighs belly button to spine tuck the chin looking down at your lap and just hang out here feel the stretch okay let's do that again back uh thumbs to that back wall as we come into our cow pose inhale to prepare exhale come into your cat's pose let's do that again inhale cow exhale cap let's do two more inhale cow

exhale cat last one warming up that spine lovely and exhale finish up your last cat pose make sure you're not holding the head up Tuck that chin one more breath and release okay we're going to move a little bit forward in our chair and I'm going to bring my right knee up and in now if this doesn't work for your knee you're going to grab behind the thigh right either it's absolutely fine so the first stretch I want you to think about crown of the head is nice and long belly is super tight we're lengthening up as we're

pulling in so I'm not leaning back does that make sense right nice long spot okay so now grab under that thigh Flex the foot and I want you to push through your foot like you're trying to touch the wall in front of you and then we're going to bring that foot down bend the knee and put the foot on the floor let's do the same side again here we go bring it in squeeze lifting up nice and Tall through the spine

Crown the head to the ceiling Flex we're going to push through the heel lengthening through that leg put that

foot on the floor bend the knee and put that foot down okay so now we're going to do the other side here we go bring it in first and squeeze so I'm just kind of squeezing pulling that knee in and lengthening through the spine remember you can always just hold right here if that feels better for you okay now let's everybody hold under the thigh Flex the foot try to touch the wall in front of you with that leg place that foot down heel down bend the knee and put the foot on the floor again bring it in squeeze

Flex lengthen push put the foot down and release okay so now we're going to do that same thing but we're we're going to hold on to the chair instead of our leg okay you'll feel the abdominals working here okay so abdominals and quadricep are going to be working pretty hard but let's hold that chair let's bring that knee up Flex push through the heel place the heel down on the floor bend the knee and put the foot down let's do the same side again bring it in Flex push through put the foot on the floor and release

other side bring that knee in Flex the foot push through the heel try to touch that wall in front of you don't lean back put the foot on the floor bend the knee let's do it again bring it in Flex push out the heel down and bend that knee okay really really good work there now we're going to do one more version of this and this is going to be with a little exterior rotation of the knee so you're going to begin to feel it a little more in the hip that one you probably felt more in the quadricep and

the hamstring right this one you're going to feel a little more in the hip okay so first thing we're going to do is bring that knee in just like we did previously but now what I'm going to do is I'm going to take my hand I'm going to place it right under my ankle do you see what's happening there rotating so I'm rotating that leg keeping the knee bent now Flex the foot if you want a little more you can hold on to that leg or if you want to try don't hold on to the chair or the leg there's the

abdominals working a little bit more do you see how I maintain that external rotation my toes are out to that side at a diagonal put the foot down bend the knee and let's do that again bring it in squeeze externally rotate Flex the foot now hold on to the leg if you want to hold on to the chair if you want to or if you're with me pull that belly in tight keep that spine long let go Flex push through that hell you see oh I've got that external rotation put that leg down bring it in last time on this side squeeze it externally rotate Flex that foot let go or hold on push place that foot down and release okay how'd that feel I feel that a nice little stretch right right out here and I'm working my abdominals let's do the other side so we're going to bring it in first ah making sure that spine is long we're pulling that knee in right belly is tight all right so now this is the hand I'm going to place under my ankle externally rotate Flex push hold on if you wish hold the chair if you wish or nothing place that foot down and release bring that knee in don't lose that external rotation right so we externally rotate here Flex now hold that external rotation toes are out to that outer corner right feeling that work there put the foot down and release one more bring it in squeeze externally rotate Flex push place the foot on the floor toes up and release how did that feel those are actually called seated lunges so really good work now I'm going to go ahead and grab my strap so again if you don't have

a strap you're going to do this you can substitute the necktie or the SCAR or if you want to just do it without it that's fine too but you'll see how the strap will help us here so I'm gonna hook this strap under right under that right i'm right foot and you want it on the ball of the foot okay so don't bring it to the arch the arch of the foot is full of really tiny bones right and so we don't want to put a lot of pressure on that but you can put the pressure on the ball of the foot okay so

here we go we've got the strap hooked under that foot now I'm going to extend my leg long so what's happened here is my arm if I were to try to do this with my hand which is technically the way this pose would be I'd be holding onto my pretty challenging right that's how very so all I've done now is with the strawberries I've just made my arm a little bit longer and it makes this pose a little more accessible for me to to maintain the proper form so you've got your neck tie strapped around or you've

got your scarf or you've got your yoga strap or you've got your hand hooked right here okay so I'm gonna let you pick the version that works for you all right so let's just give it a little tug there's a that hamstring you feel that I know I do too okay so now you're right I'm sorry your left hand you're going to grab both straps okay your other arm you can hold on to the chair if you wish or you can bring it out to the side here's the important part I'm not leaning back great so make

sure the crown of the head stays up and we're going to bring that leg across the midline of the body oh yeah you feeling that stretch right there let's come center now grab it with the right hand opposite arm extends out now look at what

I'm doing I'm opening up there's that inner thigh ha last come back Center we're going to do that again on each side um and center and then open it up let's come forward bend that knee and release okay how did that feel it's pretty good I like this this is just such a nice

stretch okay so we're going to hook the ball the strap under the ball of the foot again go ahead and lift that leg up now if you want to just hold on to one one strap in each hand and give it a little tug for the hamstring stretch go for it remember lengthen through the crown of the head I'm not leaning back right my belly is so tight here okay so now this hand I'm going to grab the strap opposite arm extends out and we'll bring that leg across the midline of the body so it's a nice stretch right here and

the other nice thing about having the strap or the neck tie or the scarf is you can change the angle of this leg right so maybe you want to bring it up a little bit higher maybe you want to bring it down a little bit lower you can choose and this gives you some options okay let's grab that strap with the other hand bring it out oh yeah are you leaning back don't don't do it let's Concentra again grab that strap open last grab the strap and open it up again the other way oh my goodness inner thighs one more breath come up bend that

knee and release okay ha everybody doing all right okay we're gonna come to standing beside our chair now so we're going to do that same pose that we just did seated but we're going to do it standing so you've got your chair here for support okay you've got that chair you can hang on to that chair so there is a little bit of balance here so what I want you to do is put the weight into the leg next to the chair okay then the other foot you're going to step into your strap alright so now with my right hand I'm going to

grab that strap I'm going to hold on one chair between my chair with my left and we'll lift that leg up hello you feeling okay so keep your abdominals engaged here nice long spine now all I'm going to do is I'm going to bring my leg across to my chair and I'm just going to set my foot right into the seat of that chair and feel that stretch notice how my hips have tried to stay forward right so I'm trying not to let my hips move with my leg okay now I'm going to bring this leg out

and then I'm going to open it up hold that chair this is not your balance don't worry about balance right now we're going to come back Center let's bring it across again make sure your abdominals are engaged though right even though I'm holding that chair I want to still have my abs engaged let's come Center out we go and center and let's release that and we're going to come to the other side so we do have one more thing we're going to add on but let's do the other side first

and then we'll add that on okay so again I've got the weight in the leg next to the chair super important that we go with the right leg the correct leg okay so now my left leg is going to step into that strap you see that this is the hand I'm going to grab those that strap I don't know I like to choke up just a little bit does that that work for you as I lift that leg up I just feel like I have a little more control all right my abdominals are engaged my spine is long crown of the head to the

ceiling let's bring that leg across and just set it in the seat of the chair feel the stretch keep those hips facing forward hi all right are we ready let's open and then we're going to open that leg up hold that chair right and then we're going to come Center then we're going to place that foot back on the chair again ah and center and let's open one more time now we're going to go ahead and add that on to this side so what I want you to do now is bend your knee leave that strap right where it is and I want you to

bring the strap up and over your shoulder oh there's that quadricep isn't it you feel that okay so this is we're moving into dancer pose so the standing knee is soft all right so I've got that sanding knee soft now here's the thing if you want to try the balance and you're going to let go of the chair if you start to fall I want you to drop the strap so I have seen this happen in my class somebody is standing here and then all of a sudden they just fall over I want you to drop the strap and put your foot down okay so

don't just drop that strap or don't do it right just keep holding onto the chair but if you want to give it a try let me get back in here I just kind of wanted to show you that whole idea of dropping that strap alright so here we go we're going to let go of the chair belly tight right balance is all about abdominals and then we're just going to extend that arm out there's your dancer pose lovely one more breath here grab the chair and release okay let's do dancer on the other side so remember we're going to stab that

right foot into the into the strap okay we're going to lift it up now all you're going to do is bend your knee and bring that strap up back and behind okay and if the the strap on the foot kind of moves to the ankle it's okay doesn't matter it doesn't have to stay on the foot it can be on the ankle okay we're holding that chair for right now we've got our abdominals as tight as we can get them we're going to let go of the chair and we're going to bring our hand up one more breath here bring that hand

back down and release very very good okay so let's just set our strap down for right now and we're going to move forward so what I want you to think about is that the arches of your feet are even with the front legs of the chair okay so I'm not back here I know everybody wants to hang on to that you'll see why here in just a minute go ahead and take a step forward okay now with this leg the leg next to the chair okay your left leg you're going to take a step back onto those toes and now see the chair is

right in the right place isn't it so you've got that chair right here to hold on to okay so now what I'd like for you to do is Bend is take your front foot and heel toe it out one time okay so what I want you to have is some space between your front foot and your back foot you're on your back toes so you're not on that that foot isn't flat you're up on those toes if that feels okay all right bend your front knee a little bit more you should be feeling quite a stretch here on this back leg

now we're going to pull our belly in really tight we're going to let go of the chair and we're going to bring our hands to Heart how does that feel anybody okay all right get your balance make sure your feet you've got space between those feet and what I call this is if you want railroad tracks not feed on a tightrope but you want your feet on railroad tracks okay so you want some space between them all right we're gonna inhale to prepare exhale we're going to bring our hands to the ceiling here we are in a beautiful

Crescent lunge now you're going to Windmill and face your chair oh there's some balance right hands to the ceiling Windmill and face the other way I know it's challenging hands to the ceiling bring your hands back to Heart grab the chair and release oh how did that feel I know so we got a bit of work going on in those legs don't we a little bit of work for the legs okay so let's do the other side so remember we now you know why I want you to start forward so when you step back you've got

that chair right in the right place so we're going to step back with the leg next to the chair okay so the right leg take that step back be up on those toes let's heel toe that front foot out a little bit right see what's happened there I'm on my back toes I'm not on my foot isn't flat this front foot is out my hips are forward and we'll bend that front knee there we go there's a beginning of a crescent lunge right belly tight let's bring our hands to heart to start see how that feels okay inhale to prepare exhale extend the arms up there's a beautiful Crescent lunge okay we're going to Windmill and face our chair we know those arms you feel it can it hands to the ceiling we're going to Windmill the other way ready we got this hands to the ceiling grab the chair and release it oh my goodness okay very very good so we're going to move into humble Warrior and I'll tell you what I'm going to do I'm gonna put we're going to come back to the strap here in just a minute

but I'm going to set it under my chair just to get it out of my way for right now so why don't you join me in doing that and that way we know we're not going to trip over it or it's not in the seat of the chair in our way okay so I'm going to turn and I'm going to face the seat of my chair now again the leg next to the back of the chair I know I'm like a harping on that but that's the one you want to take a little step under the chair so when you bend your knee you're going

to touch the chair okay so you see what's happening there mini my knee and it's touching okay so now I'm gonna take this back foot and we'll step it back now this time I'm not on my toes I've got that back foot down okay so it's at that angle so the heel is down my hips are facing the chair and I'm gonna bend my front knee we're going to move into a warrior one okay so let's go ahead and pull our belly in thinking about lengthening through the tailbone belly is tight bring your hands

to Heart okay inhale to prepare exhale we're going to hand our have our hands come up towards the ceiling for a full version of our Warrior One pose now bring your hands back behind you interlace your fingers press those fingers down towards the the floor do you see what's happening I'm lifting up my chest is opening now we're going to Bow over that front leg you want to keep that front knee bent okay so I'm bowing over that front leg and what I'm going to do is I'm going to take my outside shoulder my

left shoulder and I'm going to bring it over towards that front knee one more breath here let's take the twist out come back up to standing and let's just take a little break we're going to do that again on this side and we're going to see if maybe your forehead will come to the chair so instead of doing the crossing over you're going to stay straight and see if you can get your forehead down it doesn't matter right just I'm just giving you options I'm giving you ideas but we're going to stay on this side and

do it one more time and then we'll go to the other side okay so humble Warrior so let's do it again so we got this foot next to the back of the chair we're going to bend that knee touching bring that back foot back behind you put us at that 45 degree angle face lips face your chair bend that front knee touch that chair pull that belly in lengthen through that tailbone so my weight is back right my weight isn't up here my weight is back bring your hands to Heart okay are we ready inhale to prepare

exhale extend those arms up to the ceiling see how that feels there's our Warrior One pose now I'm going to clasp my hands behind my back interlace the fingers push those Knuckles down towards the floor see how I'm opening up through the chest front knee stays bent okay are we ready now this time as we come forward instead of bringing that shoulder across to the opposite knee we're just going to begin to let the head fall towards the chair and then the arms are going to lift up back behind you

and we just have one more breath here okay pull your belly in push through that front heel let's come back up to standing there's your power move make those legs work and release how did that feel that front leg was working hard wasn't it let's do the other side so here we are we're going to come across to the other side put that foot under make sure that when you bend the knee it touches stepping back back foot at that 45 degree angle hips are forward bend that front knee so I don't know

if you notice but see how far away I am from my chair so I was just inching my foot forward a little bit now I want to be able to touch that chair okay so this is a little adjustment that I made right hips forward bring your hands to Heart okay inhale to prepare pull that belly in lengthen through that tailbone exhale extend those arms up keep that front knee bent beautiful Warrior One pose okay we're gonna do a humble Warrior clasp your hands behind your back interlace your fingers push those Knuckles down see how I'm lifting up

through the heart now the first one when we come down I want you to take this shoulder and bring it across to that knee okay so I'm coming down I'm going to take my shoulder across my body to that bent knee and my arms are lifting up back behind me one more breath here let's go ahead and come up to standing can we just do it let's do it this one's gonna be forehead towards the chair press those Knuckles down lift through that heart squeeze those shoulder blades behind now as I come down my forehead is

going to come towards the mat my arms are coming up back behind me humble Warrior one more breath okay you're gonna push through that front heel there's your power move lift that heart up and release okay very very good work now we're going to do a warrior one but we're going to move into a pyramid pose okay so we're going to stay on this side of the chair we've got that foot under we know kind of know our Warrior one now don't we pull that belly in right lengthen through the tailbone bring your

hands to Heart stand down that back leg okay inhale here exhale extend those arms up to that Warrior one now the difference is instead of leaving that front knee bent now we're going to straighten that front leg right let's bring our hands back extend and then keep that front leg straight and then come down oh yeah there's that hamstring do you feel that now listen to my voice what I want you to do now is let go of the hands bring them into the seat of the chair okay ha how's that feel little pyramid pose

all right let's go ahead and lift up and grab that chair and let's go to the other side okay so now I've got again the leg next to the back of the chair when I'm in that knee step back on that back heel right hips are forward bend the knee touch the chair lots of stuff to remember I know but we've done this one a few times now I think we kind of got it don't we bring your hands to Heart pull that belly in lengthen through that tailbone inhale exhale extend those arms up all right now we're going to straighten

that front leg let's bring that hands back behind us lengthen nice and long keep the front leg straight come forward okay now let's let go of the of the hands and place them in the seat of our chair and just see if you can lower your heart anymore right so a little bit of triangle pose here so there's the hamstring stretching you feel that that front leg is straight my hips are forward oh that feels so good to me one more breath here and come up and release very good all right let's come back to

seated now we're going to do another uh pose with our strap if you have it if you don't have it obviously you'll do it without it it's fine but if you're with me we're going to strap that around the ball of that right foot and I'm gonna put my heels on the floor lengthen through the spine now I'm just going to walk my hands down that strap and that's just giving me a little extra stretch we're really warm so we can encourage that hamstring to open just a little bit more so this is a

seated pyramid pose we just did a standing pyramid pose now we're doing a seated pyramid pose with the strap and one more breath here and let's release that go ahead and unravel and let's do the other side ah right so we're gonna do that I'm gonna lengthen through the spine keep my back flat as I walk my hands down that strap remember the other thing too is looking out not down that's going to help you keep that back flat we want this leg straight so we're not bending the knee we're keeping the legs

straight and we're just letting that that hamstring we're giving it some love one more breath all right let's unravel the strap and we're just going to sit it down by our side now I'm going to take my ankle and we'll place it on my knee if this doesn't feel good for you for Pigeon pose you're going to stay ankle to ankle it's a great option the other thing you can do if you want a little bit more that might work is you extend your leg and then you bring that ankle up more

towards the shin okay so I've got you've got three versions here that work for you my the version I'm going to do is ankle to me okay works for me so I'm going to hang out here just for a couple of breaths now lengthening through the spine if you wish and letting that heart begin to fall forward that's going to get a little deeper into that stretch okay let's tuck the chin and roll it up and we're gonna rock our baby so I'm just going to lift my leg up and I want to move that leg back and forth so this

is for the hip joint and then I'll set that leg down and then I'm going to lengthen through the spine one more time and let my heart fall forward so one more little add-on if you like it it's just to press gently on that leg okay let's release it and we're going to go to the other side all right so remember you've got ankle to ankle is aversion you've got ankle to shin that's another version and if you're with me we're going to do ankle to knee and we're hanging out here first we're

just feeling the stretch then we're going to lengthen through the spine and begin to let the heart fall forward okay let's go ahead and lift up now lift go ahead and reach down and grab your leg and we're going to rock our baby a little side to side and then we're going to place that leg down lengthen through the spine begin to let that heart fall forward and if you want you can just press gently here ah we just have one more breath all right let's move into shavasana pose so we're going to sit back in our chair

lean back if you wish hands are going to rest lightly on your thighs flip your palms up towards the ceiling close your eyes take a deep breath in and a full breath out meaningful path with all its goings on life often seems like an intentional assault on you but that's rarely the case your best approach is not to take it personally the distractions and frustrations are just part of reality you can accept that reality with all it encompasses then you're able to keep on going in the direction of your original intent

there was a time not so long ago when you when you felt peaceful focused confident filled with purpose you were in that state and now you can get back to it again it's not as far away as it seems in fact just thinking about being more peaceful starts to get you feeling more peaceful the petty interruptions and distractions will come and go and through it all you can continue following a meaningful path know that deeply and know mere distraction will have the power to distract you for long take a deep breath in

and a full breath out drop your right ear towards your right shoulder reach up with the right hand give the head a gentle tug pressing that left hand down towards the floor release it drop your chin towards your chest reach up with your hands give the head a gentle tug release it drop your left ear towards your left shoulder reach up with the left hand give the head a gentle tug pressing that right hand down towards the floor release it look out just slightly open your mouth if you want to stretch your jaw bring your hands to your heart

DAY 19

let's get started so we're going to sit up nice and tall in our chair we're moving forward we're not leaning back taking a moment to focus on that mind and body and breath we're going to ground those feet to the Earth we're going to ground our sits bones to the chair let's lift our heart lower our shoulders out of the ears place your hands lightly on your thighs flip those Palms up close your eyes and connect to your heart center let go of everything outside of the room focusing your attention inward let's begin to notice the breath your natural inhalation and exhalation and then we're going to elongate that

breath so we're going to inhale a little more deeply and exhale a little more completely let's do that again inhale and exhale this time try to make that exhalation longer than the inhalation inhale and exhale and breathe normally bring your hands to your heart set your intentions for today's practice one more breath here bring your hands back down to your thighs and open your eyes we're going to bring our hands down by our side and we're going to shrug our shoulders up into our ears and then we're going to let them fall

let gravity help there let's shrug those shoulders up into the ears and then let them fall let's do that one more time shrug those shoulders and let them fall let's move to a extended Mountain so we're going to lengthen our arms up towards the ceiling remember pull the shoulders down belly is tight we're going to lean our Mountain just a little bit here super gentle thinking about keeping this hip down and we're going to bring those hands up and we're going to lean our Mountain the

other way and come up and bring your hands down and just take a little break okay so we're going to do that again adding on we're going to bring our palms together interlace our fingers and have our pointer finger to the ceiling okay so let's do that again let's do that extending those arms up to the ceiling Palms are together interlace your fingers pointer finger is up to the ceiling okay now we're going to lean our Mountain again remember keeping the the hip down right this opposite hip stays down

okay let's come up and we're going to lean the other way and we're going to come up now let's lean again and then I want you just to turn and look up at the ceiling so just a little gentle twist here take the twist out come up and we're going to lean the other way gentle twist up and release that hands back to the ceiling and release all right excellent work so we're going to do some full body circles then we're going to start by just leaning to the left hands are on those thighs we're

going to come forward hold on to those thighs give yourself a little support then we're going to come to the right now as we go back we're going to try to lean back as far as we can without resting on that chair you'll feel your abdominals engaged and then let's do that again so we're just making a big circle here there's your back there's your other side and then now let's all come back up to seated and we're going to do that again but we're going to reverse it all right so we're

going to start to the right this time and then let's go forward to the left and back let's do that again full body circles just a little warm up for the spine belly stays tight and let's come up to seated okay so now the add-on for that one I call stirring the pot so we're going to use our arms and we're acting like we're stirring a big cauldron okay so we're going to be engaging our arms we're going to get a little deeper into that back and a little bit more into those core muscles

so if you want to do the previous version it's fine you don't ever have to add on ever but if you want to add on we're going to grab that stick and we're going to come forward there's your back working belly tight let's come to the right and back we go there's your abdominals come to the left make that Circle let's do that again okay and it's going to reverse it one more time and release all right excellent work just warming up through the center of the body right a little bit of that core

warm up okay so we're going to do a variation on horse pose if you've been with me through this series we have done horse pose before this was just a little bit different so the first thing we're going to do is we're going to lift our right heel up off the mat okay and then we're going to put that heel down and then we're going to lift the left heel up and we're going to put it down let's do that again lift and down and lift and down again lift down lift down last one lift down lift and down okay so now there's gonna

be a little brain work so my right heel is going to lift but my left toes are going to lift so we call this rocking and now they're both uh both feet are flat and then we're reversing it so one heel in the other toes and feet are flat and Rock you feel it and flat and Rock and flat and Rock last one last side we've got this and release a little movement for those feet should feel like a really good stretch now the first add-on is going to be an arm lift and remember you don't have to do the arm you know you don't have to add on but I'm going to go back to the heel and the same arm of the heel that's lifting is I'm lifting that arm and then I'm going to come down and then the other side lift and down switch lift and down again lift and down lift down lift and down okay so the final add-on is instead of the heel I'm going to lift the knee and the arm same side here we go lift and down breathe and switch sides lift and down let's switch lift and down and switch lift and down again lift is your abdominals tight right or your belly

button to spine we just do one more on each side keeping the back nice and long crown of the head to the ceiling and release all right good work there okay so now we're going to start with just a half shoulder press I'm going to start again with my right arm and it's just a half shoulder press okay and let's do that again just see how that feels and then we're going to come down and let's do the other side so I want you to just check in with those shoulders see how that's feeling okay now let's go to the other side and

we're going to the half shoulder press and then we're going to open and then we're going to college what are we working on right you feel that shoulder uh that joint there let's lift and open and close and down let's do that again lift and open close and down other side lift open close and down okay we've got one more thing to add so we're going to do the half shoulder press we're going to open Close turn your palm to face you and then do a bicep curl let's do that other side half shoulder

press up open and bicep curl okay so now checking in how's everything feeling right I know it's a lot of work on that joint that shoulder joint we want to keep those joints nice and movable right mobile I guess that's the right word okay so we can do both at the same time so we're going to start with that half shoulder press we're going to open we're going to close both hands do a bicep curl and then we're going to do that again oops I forgot the shoulder press and then open and then bicep curl now the final add-on

if your shoulders are feeling okay Palms face each other you're going to do a full press all the way to the ceiling and down and open and close bicep curl let's do that again Palms face each other shoulder press all the way to the ceiling and down open your book and close bicep curl let's do one more just one more press it Up full shoulder press and open Palms face you bicep curl and release how did that feel I know a little bit of work on those shoulders okay we're going to come to standing behind our chair all right so this is a standing pigeon pose now you're going to stay behind your chair and you've got to have that chair right there for support I'm just going to step out so you can see me a little bit better but you stay right behind that chair so I'm stepping out just a little bit so you can see me so we're going to put our weight into our left leg and we're going to cross ankle to ankle okay pull your belly in super tight push your hips back all right so just hold on hanging onto the back of that chair now

if if it's in your way you can step back a little bit if that makes sense right if the back of the chair is kind of in your way so it would be here you could always step back just a little bit so I'm crossing at the ankles my hips are shooting back standing pigeon pose and let's come up and we're going to go straight to the other side for this one okay before we add on so we're going to cross ankle to ankle you can bend the supporting knee a little bit shoot your hips back that's the key to

this whole series is making sure those hips shoot back and then let your heart fall so the the sensation is back here okay so the stretch is happening in that glute area Okay one more breath and come up okay so now what I'd like for you to think about is walking your hands down the sides of the chair okay so you'll be Crossing let's go back to the other side which one did we do I think we had the I don't remember it doesn't matter we're gonna do both so I'm going to take my left leg

and I'm going to cross it in front I'm going to bend my supporting knee I'll shoot my hips back now if it feels okay what you'll do is you'll begin to walk your hands down the back of the chair and you continue to shoot your hips back oh my how does that feel do you feel that right here in this glute I do okay we have one more breath and let's come up and let's switch sides okay so the other weight is in the other leg cross at the ankle bend that supporting knee just a little bit right belly stays tight now as you

begin to bend a supporting knee push your hips back behind you and begin to let that heart fall forward walking the hands down the back of your chair you've got that support this is not balance hang on to that chair is fine let's do one more breath and then we're going to come up and release okay now this is this is a significant add-on so I want you to just do what works for you if you want to stick with this version Crossing ankle to ankle please do hold the chair if you want to try the next version I'm going to bend my

supporting knee just a little bit and then I'm going to bring that leg up above that knee so I'm bending the knee to kind of give this ankle a spot to sit right does that make sense okay hang out here first how's that feeling I know right here this is what you should be feeling this hip and blue hang on to that chair all right bend that supporting knee shoot the hips back move your hands down the chair if that feels okay maybe you even bring your hands down to the seat of the chair how does that feel

oh yeah we have one more breath all right let's all come back up to standing mark it out just a little bit and we're going to go to the other side let's do it so standing knee is soft Crossing that ankle up above it so we be sure you've got that little spot for that ankle to hang out here okay are you feeling it bend that supporting knee shoot the hips back behind you and maybe you begin to walk your hands down that chair the back of the chair maybe even to the seat of the chair oh boy that's quite a stretch

we have one more breath here and up we got all right let's take a moment here and walk that out that's really really good work I feel that right through here right good stretch okay we're going to move into a standing tree pose so we've got our hands right here on that chair and I want you to put the weight into the leg next to the chair okay and then we're going to create our kickstand so this heel is just up against the ankle of the standing foot okay does that make sense you feel that all right so balance this is a balanced

pose and remember balance poses require us to really focus in on the abdominals so we pull that belly in we lift those pelvic floor muscles up like just really engaging all of these muscles here find a spot that's not moving it really helps if you kind of focus in on some area in front of you we're going to let go of that chair and we're going to bring our hands to our heart see how that feels belly tight okay now inhale to prepare from here and then we're just going to add our branches to our trees hands to the

ceiling beautiful chair pose tree pose one more breath here let's bring your hands back down to the chair and release okay very very good so we're going to do the other side we're going to come to the other side of our chair we're going to place the weight into the leg next to the chair and we're going to create that kickstand okay so my heel is just kind of resting up against the ankle of that standing leg I've got my hand on that chair I'm going to pull that belly in as tight as I can I'm going to lift those pelvic

floor muscles I'm going to lower my shoulders out of my ears find that spot that's not moving focus in on it bring your hands to your heart and how to prepare we're going to add the branches to our trees we have one more breath bring your hands back down and release that's so good good good good good okay so we're going to come back behind our chair and we're going to work into a goddess pose so from here we're going to do a heel toe heel toe so my knees that are in alignment with my toes and my toes are out at a

diagonal barely stays tight let's go ahead and hold that chair for right now bend your knees now your hips are going to go back okay so what I don't want to have happen let me just show you stay behind your chair so what I don't want to have happen is when you bend your knees your knees come forward that's not what I don't want your knees in front of your toes okay so as you bend your knees you're shooting your hips back you should feel your quadriceps working okay belly tight all right Are We There are we feeling

okay all right so now what we're going to do is we're going to let go of that chair let's take our left hand first and place it on our belly and take our other hand and place it on our heart let's take a deep breath in here see if you can feel your belly extend as you inhale and exhale again inhale and exhale one more inhale place your hands on that chair straighten the legs and let's come back in and take a break okay we're going to do that again and what I'd like for you to see is if you

can get a little deeper into squat okay into that goddess pose just see if it works for you okay let's start here with that heel toe heel toe make sure your toes are at a diagonal we're going to pull that belly in super tight lift those pelvic floor muscles we're going to bend our knees and shoot our hips back hold that chair is fine can you get any deeper into your goddess paths okay let's take the other hand to the belly and the opposite hand to the heart let's take a deep breath in feel that belly extend exhale pull that

belly button in let's do that again inhale and exhale let's do one more inhale and exhale place your hands on the chair straighten those legs and heel toe those feet back together excellent work let's come back to seated so I'm forwarding my chair I'm not leaning back let's take our right knee and open let your left knee fall down towards the floor turn so that you're facing this wall so you're up on those back toes this back leg is nice and long maybe you extend the kneecap back of the kneecap

towards the ceiling for a little more stretch here you feel that Crescent lunge and release it and let's do that one more time oh yeah feeling that stretch one more breath let's release that and face forward same leg extend it out in front of you toes to the ceiling lengthen through the spine belly tied hands on thighs moving into pyramid pose looking out beyond your toes not look down tuck the chin and roll it up inhale extend exhale come forward tuck that chin and roll it up we've got one more inhale nice and long exhale

forward we go and Tuck that chin and roll it up same leg we're going to bring it either onto that knee if that feels okay for you or you're going to cross at the ankle either is fine lengthen nice and long through the spine on an inhale exhale keep the back flat looking out not down and let that heart begin to fall forward tuck that chin and roll it up inhale to prepare exhale down we go high and roll it up last one inhale exhale down we go and release let's place that foot on the floor and we're going to go to the other

side let's open nice and wide first we're going to let this knee fall down towards the floor push that foot back behind you and lift that heart up maybe back in the kneecap lengthens up towards the ceiling hold and breathe your crescent lunge hold the movement not the breath release it let's do that one more time and release go ahead and face forward extend the same leg out in front of you toes up to the ceiling hands resting on the thighs extend through the spine on an inhale exhale let that heart fall

forward pyramid pose tuck that chin and roll it up extend nice and long inhale exhale down we go look out not down one more tuck that chin and roll it up exhale down we go and roll it up okay ready for Pigeon remember ankle to ankle is an option or ankle to knee your choice nice long spine inhale exhale let that heart fall forward lookout tuck the chin and roll it up inhale to prepare exhale down we go wow I feel this one a lot and Tuck that chin and roll it up do you find one side more willing than the other right

down we go oh yeah and release okay we made it move it moving into shavasana pose so let's just move back in our chair leaning back if that feels okay for you hands resting lightly on the thighs flip the Palms up to the ceiling close your eyes take a deep breath in and a full breath out activate your resourcefulness some people have access to great and varied resources others have a characteristic that can be even more valuable resourcefulness no matter what you have or don't have you can find ways to make better use of

it by employing your resourcefulness and learning from the experience you strengthen that resourcefulness resourcefulness is a child of gratitude the more appreciative you are for whatever you have the more ways you can find to make good use of it without sufficient resourcefulness time resources and opportunities give get wasted that doesn't do any good a life of fulfillment is not primarily about what you start with it's more about what you do with it how can you make use of what's available to get from where you are to where you

desire allow gratitude to activate your resourcefulness and you're well on the way take a deep breath in and a full breath out drop your right ear towards your right shoulder reach up with the right hand give the head a gentle tug pressing that left hand down towards the floor release it drop your chin towards your chest reach up with your hands give the head a gentle tug release it drop your left ear towards your left shoulder reach up with the left hand give the head a gentle tug pressing that right hand down towards the floor release it look up just slightly open your mouth if you want to stretch your jaw bring your hands to your heart.

Please wait, Your Review is Very Important…

Dear Reader,

I hope this message finds you well. Thank you for choosing to read the 28 Day Chair Yoga for Seniors to Lose Weight. Your feedback is incredibly valuable to me, and I would love to hear your thoughts on the book. Whether you've just started, are halfway through, or have finished reading, your perspective matters.

Your feedback is immensely appreciated and will help me enhance future works.

Thank you for taking the time to share your thoughts on 28 Day Chair Yoga for Seniors to Lose Weight. Your support means the world to me.

Happy reading!

Carol Bolden

DAY 20

let's get started we're going to sit up nice and tall in our chair we have moved forward we're not leaning back taking that moment to focus on the mind and the body and the breath placing both feet on the floor and grounding each foot grounding those sits bones to the seat of the chair lift your heart lower your shoulders down out of the ears place your hands lightly on your thighs lift the Palms up to the ceiling close your eyes and connect to your breath we're going to move that breath down into the diaphragm as you inhale the belly extends we're filling the lungs from the bottom up and as you exhale pull the belly button

in towards the spine push the air up and out of the lungs do that again breathe normally we're going to continue with that diaphragmatic breath and we're going to inhale to four counts exhale to five something like this inhale two three four exhale two three four five inhale two three four exhale two three four five and breathe normally bring your hands to your heart set your intentions for today's practice one more breath bring your hands down to your thighs and open your eyes we're going to roll our shoulders

up back and down okay so take your time here right forward and up and back and then let's reverse them so we're going back first and then up and then forward and down do that again oh yeah that should feel really really good okay and let's release that excellent we're going to move into pelvic tilt so we're going to take our pointy pit bones here right here on the pelvis you got these really pointy bones we're going to rock those towards our shoulders so see what's happening I've

got a little I'll show you from the side so it's a little pelvic tilt right now we're going to take those hip tips and rock them towards our our knees and then kind of lift up see what's happening there let's do that again hip tips to shoulders and hit tips to knees and again pelvic tilts so rocking forward and back a little warm up for that spine let's do that one more time and re-release okay very good so my feet are on the floor and I'm going to reach back and I'm going to hold the chair and I want you to think

about nice long spine belly is tight and then I'm going to take my feet just a little bit wider than hip distance okay so not quite you know together but not like goddess either hold that the chair and then let your knees fall to the right and then come up and then we're going to let our knees fall the other way so I'm kind of coming up onto the edges of my feet right so if that feels okay for you and then come Center okay so we're just going to do one add-on here so we're going to let our knees fall to

the right and then I want you to look over the opposite shoulder make sure those shoulders are down and then we're going to bring everything Center and then we're going to do the other side just one more breath here and come Center and release that okay that should a little warm up for those legs should have felt really really good now I'm going to move forward in my chair the next pose is called Bada konasana it's bound angle pose cobbler pose it's got a few different names so what I want you to do is you've got

your hands on your thighs and then I want to put the soles of my feet together do you see kind of what I'm doing there I don't know if you can see that very clearly my knees are wide the soles of my feet are together my hands are just going to rest here on my thighs okay so if this is if you're feeling a little unstable on the chair you can always go ahead and hold the chair and that's fine if you don't want to just have your hands on the thighs we're going to lengthen through the spine pull

the belly in and we're going to begin to let that heart fall forward ah right one more breath here and we're going to roll roll up into a seated position and we're going to do that one more time nice long spine belly tight let that heart fall forward hold on to that chair is fine right I'm going to hold on to my chair this time I think so the more that you can keep the back flat and look out not down is where you're going to maximize that stretch right so we're all about optimizing the stretch tuck the

chin and roll it up and we're just going to do that one final time inhale extend exhale come forward oh that feels good one more breath tuck that chin roll it up place your feet on the floor ah so we're going to move into seated camel pose now you're going to be lifting up sitting up nice and tall in your chair nice long spine and now what I'm going to do is I'm going to place one hand on each side of my spine right in the small of my back you stay facing forward I'm going to turn to the side just so you

can see me a little better so see I've got one hand right in the small of the back on each side and now all I'm going to do my feet are on the floor all I'm going to do is I'm going to push my hips forward so as I push my hips forward do you see what's happening there's just a little bitty arch in the back and see if that feels okay for you okay now I'm going to release that I'm going to pull my belly in and then I'm going to round into a cat pose place your hands on those thighs now I'm going

to Face Forward place your hands on the thighs elbows are wide pull your belly in and round down okay so we're going to come back up into seated position so let's do that again before we add on so we're going to place our hands right in the small of the back push those hips forward lifting up just thinking about lifting just a little bit right maybe opening up a little bit through the throat that's all feeling that more of a push forward than anything a little arch in the back you feel that little camel pose

okay now pull the belly in we're going to move into cat pose just to release that okay so elbows are wide hands are on those thighs and we're tucking our chin and letting the head fall rounding that spine into our cat pose okay so now if you want just a little bit more you're going to push the hips forward a little bit I want you to lift up through the chest and squeeze your shoulder blades behind if that doesn't feel good on your back don't do it right it's okay just you can keep doing the previous version or don't

do any of them but if you're with me my hands are going to be back in the small of my back one on each side of my spine push those hips forward okay so this is kind of where we've been before now I want you to think about lifting through the chest opening up maybe look up squeeze your shoulder blades behind you and see if you can push those hips forward anymore just a little bit more of a back arch one more breath and let's come down into cat pose we're just going to do that one more time all right here we go

camel pose push those hips forward looking up squeeze your shoulder blades behind you if that feels okay one more breath here and then we're going to round down into that cat pose and release okay excellent work all right we're going to come to standing on the right side of our chair now we're going to add on from yesterday's tree pose if you were with me yesterday we started in tree with our kickstand and then that's pretty much what we did and we're just going to build a little bit more into our tree pose and we're

going to add a warrior three so my weight is going into the leg next to the chair and I'm going to create my kickstand again so my heel is right up against that standing ankle I'm holding on to that chair my belly is super tight here remember key to balance is right through that stabilization happening through the core of the body right so belly type pelvic floor muscles lift okay so now let's just do kickstand to start with I'm going to let go of the chair I'm going to bring my hands to

Heart shoulders are down out of the ears I'm going to take a deep breath in and then as I exhale I'm going to bring my hands up to the ceiling so there I'm adding my branches to my tree one more breath here bring your hands back down to your heart and release okay so now we're gonna go on to the add-ons on this side of the chair and then we'll do the whole thing on the other side okay so the first thing we're going to do is add a leg we're going to lift our foot up off of the floor so instead of having our toes down for kickstand we're going to lift our leg up now do you want to just lift your leg to your calf that's absolutely fine if you want to lift your leg up to your thigh that's absolutely fine I don't care it doesn't matter to me so you pick the version that you want to do so when we get there you'll know which one you want to do all right so remember belly tight let's create our kickstand to start with okay pull that belly in pelvic floor muscles lift look and find that spot that's not

moving we're going to let go of that chair we're going to bring our hand to our heart all right now if you want you're going to lift your leg up you can stay in kickstand if you prefer okay we're going to inhale to prepare and then we're going to add our branches to our trees I know it's very challenging I know okay bring your hands back to your heart now keep this knee lifted and I want you to bring the knee forward in front of you push your foot back behind you for warrior three prayer hands

we just have one more breath here let's bring that knee up and then we're going to put that foot on the floor and release okay so come to the other side so we want to get out of our balance poses mindfully right so we don't want to just fall out of it we want to put that foot down on purpose okay so we're going to put the weight into the leg next to the chair and we're going to create that kickstand again pull that belly in super tight find that spot that's not moving focus on it and bring your hands to Heart

ah alright are we ready let's take a deep breath in to prepare and then as we exhale we're going to lift that foot up off of the floor remember staying in kickstand is always an option let's add our branches to our trees oh so pretty all right bring your hands back to heart now we're going to move into that Warrior three pose so all you do is you bring your knee forward push that foot back behind you so this is Warrior three with prayer hands heart is lifted now the hips are square so we the hip of

the leg that's in the air we tend to want to hike it up don't let yourself do that belly tight one more breath here now we're going to come out of it mindfully we're going to bring that knee up and then we're going to put that foot on the floor with intention right on purpose I call it all right very very good so we're going to turn and face the seat of our chair we're going to move into a standing camel we did a seated camel just a minute ago and now we're going to do a standing camel

all right so my feet or hip distance apart I'm going to pull my belly in really tight I'm going to place one hand on each side of my spine just like we did seated exactly the same all right so lifting up nice and tall push forward so all I'm doing is pushing my hips forward just a little bit so I'm creating a little arch in the back how's that feel just one more breath now pull your belly in tight protect that low back come up we're going to place our hands in the seat of the chair so I'm just hanging forward

all right now I'm going to bring my shoulders over my wrists and I'm going to drop my belly and lift my heart into a cow pose and then I'm gonna pull my belly button to my spine round my shoulders into a cat pose and let's do that again drop the belly lift the heart cow pose pull the belly button in round the spine tuck that chin into cat pose bend the knees and then roll up slowly into standing okay we're going to do that again so here I am I've got my hands here on each side of my spine

right in the small in the back right we're going to push those hips forward now if it feels okay and you're like yeah this is not not so much I'm I'm doing good I'm feeling okay then I want you to lift your head a little higher looking up open up through the throat squeeze your shoulder blades back behind you creating a little bit more of a back bend but you have to listen to your body and only do what feels good for you we have one more breath here belly tight pull that belly in we're going to round

it down and we're going to come back into our cat and cow super gentle here place the hands in the seat of the chair bring the weight forward drop the belly lift the heart lift the hips into cow pose inhale if you want to add the breath exhale as you come into cat's pose and we're going to do that again inhale into cow and exhaling the cat bend your knees and roll up into a standing position okay very good so we're going to move into a warrior one we're going to do a little flow here a warrior one Warrior Two and triangle so

the leg next to the back of the chair is the one that I'm going to put my foot under so that when I bend my knee I can feel the seat of the chair opposite leg is going to step back my heel is down my foot is at a bit of an angle okay bring those hips around bend your front knee bring your hands to Heart okay so belly is tight lengthening through the tailbone inhale to prepare exhale bring your hands to the ceiling there's our Warrior One pose now starting with this outside hand I'm going to Windmill around into that

Warrior Two so my front knee is still bent my ribs are in the center of the body my belly is tight my arms are parallel to the mat let's look over those front fingertips let's flip that Palm up and back we're going to reverse our Warrior we're going to come back to that Warrior Two now we're going to straighten the front leg your upper body only is going to swing over towards the chair you see that this hip is hiking up we're going to come over the chair and we're going to come over the chair then we're going to take

this hand into the seat of the chair and lift up into our triangle pose front knee is straight you should be feeling the inner thigh of that front leg pretty substantially so the other thing I want you to think about is the hand that's in the airless everybody place it on our waist and lift our heart up a little bit more then extend okay one more breath here now I'm going to take my hand off of the chair and I'm going to come up into an X my arms are coming up into an X now I'm going to bend my front knee back

to that Warrior too and I'm going to round down into that Warrior one and I'm going to move to that Warrior too I'm going to reverse my warrior up and back and I'm going to come back to my Warrior Two straighten your front leg upper body over the chair over the chair over the chair hand down into that chair lift that heart up one more breath keep the front leg straight press arms up into an X bad to that Warrior too moved to that Warrior one back to our Warrior Two reverse up and back back to Warrior Two

straighten your front leg upper body over the chair moving into that triangle pose hand comes down to the chair lifting up one more breath here are we ready keep the front leg straight press up into that X bend that front knee and release that was quite a flow wasn't it now we get to do the other side we we're going to sit down after this though so that leg goes under the chair remember the foot's right under it so that when you bend that knee it touches opposite leg steps back hips are forward bend the front knee bring your belly in

lengthen through that tailbone bring your hands to Heart okay ha here we go inhale to prepare exhale hands to the ceiling for that beautiful Warrior one inhale to prepare exhale move to your Warrior Two flip that front Palm up and back as we reverse our Warrior we're going to come back to our Warrior Two straighten your front leg upper body over the chair over the chair over the chair hand comes down into that seat of that chair heart is lifted now from here leave that front leg straight we're going to lift the upper

body come into that X now bend that front knee into that Warrior Two move back to your Warrior one and move to your Warrior Two reverse that Warrior up and back back to Warrior Two straighten the front leg coming into triangle pose upper body comes over the chair it comes over the chair it comes over the chair that hand comes down into the chair lifting up keep that front leg straight we're going to take that hand out of the chair come into an X bend that front knee Warrior Two down and around to Warrior one

rotate to Warrior Two flip that Palm up and back reverse Warrior fight to Warrior Two straighten your front leg upper body over the chair over the chair over the chair hand down to the seat of the chair and lift up keep the front leg straight press up into that X bend the knee to Warrior Two and release excellent work whoa that was quite a little flow there wasn't it let's come back to seated ah alright very very good so the next pose is half lord of the fishes so we're going to take our right knee and we're

going to open it nice and wide okay so feel a little inner thigh stretch here to begin with then we're going to take our left arm we're going to open it wide we're going to bring it all the way across our body grab that chair crown of the head lifts turn and look over the back of your chair let's release that now make sure this knee doesn't fold in bring it across again grab the seat of the chair lengthen and twist and release okay let's do the other side so that left knee is going to open wide

that right arm is going to open first it's going to come across the body grab the chair crown of the head lifts turn look over the back of your chair let's release that and we're going to do that one more time bring it across that body grab the chair lift and twist making sure that this knee doesn't fold in right all right excellent work go ahead and face forward so now I'm going to take my right either ankle deck or moving into pigeon pose it can be ankle to ankle it can be ankle to knee right if you've been with me

through this journey you know the choices alright this is a good one it's one we do a lot so extend nice and long through the spine and let that heart fall forward looking out not down right tuck the chin and roll it up and we're going to do that one more time nice long spine inhale tip repair exhale as we come out and down all right and roll it up okay let's go to the other side so take your time here nice long spine inhale exhale we're going to let that heart fall forward remember pressing

gently on this knee is an option as well just giving you choices right there all of them are good and roll it up and then we're gonna do that one more time nice long spine heart Falls forward keeping the back flat and re-release all right let's move into shavasana pose we're gonna lean back if you wish hands are going to rest lightly on those thighs flip the Palms up towards the ceiling close the eyes let's take a deep breath in and a full breath out Beyond frustration frustration can put you in a foul mood

and ruin your effectiveness but it doesn't have to you can notice your frustration learn from it take positive action based on it you don't have to let it become an excuse on its own whatever is frustrating you is not forcing you to be one way or another the source of frustration may be out of your control yet your own response is very much up to you don't let frustration goat you into needless anger rudeness or other disruptive behavior instead see it as a prompt to reaffirm your own positive direction

whether your frustration is with yourself or with your situation there's nothing to be gained by perpetuating it make it your choice to move quickly beyond that frustration don't allow frustration to make you into someone you would not want to be rise above it and commit yourself once again to living at your very best take a deep breath in and a full breath out drop your right ear towards your right shoulder reach up at the right hand give the head a gentle tug pressing that left hand down towards the floor

release it drop your chin towards your chest reach up with the hands give the head a gentle tug release it drop your left ear towards your left shoulder reach up with your left hand give the head a gentle tug pressing that right hand down towards the floor release it look out just slightly open your mouth if you want to stretch your jaw bring your hands to your heart

DAY 21

we're going to move forward in our chair we're going to have our hands resting lightly on the thighs and flip those Palms up connecting to our body mind and breath grounding our feet to the Earth founding our sits bones to the chair let's lift our heart lower our shoulders out of the ears close the eyes and connect to that breath so we're feeling that natural inhalation and exhalation and then let's elongate the breath inhaling a little more deeply exhaling a little more completely do that a couple more times and release

bring your hands to your heart and set your intentions for today's practice just one more breath here bring your hands down to your thighs and open your eyes so we're going to do another breathing exercise so it bottoms down chair yoga we often will use the breath it's called uwaji and I'm sorry I said that wrong I you know what I learned duwaji and it's just one of those things that's really hard for me to correct myself but anyways it is called we and it involves breathing inhaling and

exhaling through the nose and then the other idea in that breath is that we engage our diaphragm which we talk about a lot I know I go into that diaphragm a lot and also those intercostal muscles now if you play a wind instrument or if you sing in a choir you know all about diaphragmatic breathing right we've learned that we learned that really early on as we begin to play an instrument but if you haven't done that and you really don't know what diaphragmatic breathing is all about if you'll just

simply lie down on your back and breathe you'll see the rise and fall of your belly right the belly will rise as you inhale the lungs are filling with air and then it drops as you exhale that's that diaphragm working that inhale and exhale it's also getting some assistance with those intercostal muscles which are the ones right between the ribs so to begin let's just take a deep breath in through our nose and feel the air as it passes across your throat let's do that and now as you exhale I also want you to

Exhale through the nose and feel that air crossing the throat again so let's do that again inhale exhale do that one more time inhale and exhale okay and then just breathe normally so you're feeling the air going in and out of the nose and across the throat so we're going to do that same thing but we're going to try to move the breath down into our diaphragm so instead of keeping that breath up in the chest we're going to try to get it down here into the belly okay so let's do that inhale through the nose

see if you can extend that belly and feel that belly breath and then exhale pull the belly in exhale out through the nose do that again inhale one more inhale exhale and then breathe normally okay so the very final thing we're going to do there is we're going to try to make our exhalation longer than our inhalation I'm not going to count because sometimes it can make you dizzy and I don't want anything to make you dizzy so if you're inhaling and exhaling and trying to add in the diaphragm and trying to count it

might be a little too much so I just want you to try to make that exhalation a little longer than the inhalation just at your own pace go ahead and do that a couple of times and breathe normally so sometimes we even make noise I don't know if you could hear me through the the microphones but I was making a lot of noise as I inhale and exhale and that's very common in that ujali breath okay excellent work well we're going to move on now into a wrist stretching Series so I'm going to place my hands in my lap

all right and then I'm going to interlace my fingers now I'm going to bring my arms up and I want you to press the Palms out and away from you feel that a little stretch now I'm going to lengthen my hands up towards the ceiling and then we're going to lean so it's a little bit like leaning Mountain isn't it it's very much like Lenny mountain and then up we go and then we're gonna lean the other way and then we're going to come up we're going to bring those arms out we're going to bring them down and our

palms are going to be facing up in our lap again okay so I want you to look at which pinky finger is on bottom okay and I want you to interlace your fingers the other way and it feels weird okay so my hands are resting in the uh my lap now I'm going to bring my arms up and I'm gonna press those arms away I know it feels weird it's okay let's take our hands to the ceiling and then we're going to lean our Mountain again and up and lean and up when you bring those arms out and we're going to bring them down and that

Palms are going to face up okay let's take it out and just shake those hands just for a little bit okay so the next one is going to be riding the wave so we're going to interlace our fingers the way you want to and then see what I'm doing I'm bending one elbow I mean a wrist excuse me and then the other wrist to kind of see what's happening there and then I'm going to do the other side so it's just kind of riding the way there's no real correct way to do this we're just feeling our

uh wrists kind of you know stretching and and then we're going to go the other way nice again don't worry too much about exactly what it looks like it's just the idea is stretching into those wrists and release all right very good so we're going to bring our Arms by our side and I want you to make just a really light first now I want you to rotate your wrists up towards your body as really it's kind of more of a fist isn't it and then we're going to take the fists down and then we're going to

rotate out do you see what I'm doing there and down let's bring those in and down and out and down we're going to do that one more time in and down and out and down and release okay now let's bring our arms out front make that light Fist and then we're just going to rotate to One Direction and the other direction and let's do that again just a little rotation there up and the other way and release so we're going to have our palms together right here in front now I'm calling this open the book so the pinky

finger is going to be your hinge so you're going to open your book your palms are facing you I'm hinging right at those pinky fingers now the backs of the hands are going to be together and I'm going to rotate so that my fingertips are pointing in towards my body now my fingertips are going to point down towards the floor then they're going to point out away from me now they're going to go back down towards the floor they're going to come towards my body and then I'm going to rotate right hinge up the pinky fingers

and bring the Palms together now I'm going to do that again but I'm going to hinge up the thumbs instead of the pinky fingers see what I'm doing there then I'm going to bring the backs of the hands together fingertips point away from me finger pins finger point down and then towards my body and if you can go up go up don't feel like you have to and then rotate back towards my body down towards the floor out away come up hinge at the thumbs bring the Palms together and release all right so good wrist

rotation there right shake it out a little bit all right let's take this hand I'm just all I'm going to do is I'm going to grab gently and I'm going to pull on the palm of that hand and feel a nice little stretch let's release it and we're going to do that again a nice little stretch here release and we're just going to do the other side ah this is just a very gentle pull I'm not pulling hard on that and release it and one more time it's a little stretch again for the wrist

and release okay very very good so now we're going to do Eagle arms so I'm going to bring my arms to the side my Palms are facing out okay now I want to cross my right arm on top so I've got one elbow on top of the other elbow and I'm going to bounce three times now I'm going to bend in my elbows and I'm going to bring the backs of my Palms together okay lift up now if you can bring the fronts of the Palms together go forward if that's too much for Youth and then don't stay with backs of the hands together

again we're going to lift up and we're going to bring those forearms away from our body now I'm going to twist to the left and I'm going to come Center and I'm going to twist to the right and I'm going to come Center and I'm going to unravel and take a little break okay I know that's pretty intense so remember you can always just do backs of hands together it's fine all right out we go now this time that left arm is going to be on top so you've got one elbow on top of the other you're going to bend your

elbows maybe the backs of the hands are together lift up maybe the fronts of the hands are together can you lift any higher forearms away from the face we're going to turn to the right and we're going to face Center we're going to turn to the left and we're going to face Center and we're going to unravel those arms and maybe give those shoulders a little roll all right very very good so the next thing is called Namaste hands behind the back so we're going to take our right arm it doesn't matter

and we're going to take this arm we're going to the Palm is going to face back so you're bending at the elbow see it's a little hinge here and you're going to place that hand right behind your back now the other hand the same thing Palm faces back you've got a little hinge happening here right then you're going to place that hand back behind you I'm going to turn so you can see what I'm doing behind my back now I'm going to make a little steeple see I've got my fingertips together and

I'm going to press my hands up and maybe bring those Palms together so Namaste hands but behind the back I know right it's a good stretch I'm feeling that stretch in those upper arms my chest is open I have one more breath here and let's release that roll those shoulders again we're only doing that one once okay very good so I'm going to take my right knee and I'm going to open it wide and then I'm going to bring my left knee and I'm going to bring it to meet the other leg and I'm facing the opposite wall

so my legs are facing towards a wall bring your hands up to the ceiling now starting with this outside hand you're going to Windmill around and face me okay we're going to bring those hands up to the ceiling and then we're going to Windmill around and we're going to face the back of our chair then we're going to bring those hands up and we're going to do that again windmill around and face me make sure those hips stay facing forward and up we go you should feel a good stretch into the side waist

windmilling and looking over the back of the chair fingertips to the ceiling bring the hands down and release okay let's face forward is that okay all right we're going to do the other side now so we're going to take that left knee and we're going to open it nice and wide bring that right knee around so now I'm facing the other side hands to the ceiling Windmill and face me hands to the ceiling Windmill and face over the back of your chair hands to the ceiling Windmill and face me make sure those hips and knees are

facing forward hands to the ceiling last time windmill and face over the back of your chair has to the ceiling bring the hands down to your lap and face forward okay so the next thing we're going to do is a child's pose and then the two add-ons in our child's pose is a forward fold and a rag doll so I'm here to tell you right now if those two don't work for you then you're going to stick with child's pose it is fine okay so we're going to take our feet a little bit wide because we're going to have we

need to have a spot for our body to hang out your hands are going to be Palms facing down your forearms are just going to rest here on your thighs you're going to kind of round your upper back let the head fall between your legs so this is child's pose we have one more breath now we're going to roll it up into a seated position and take just a moment so how did that feel so the idea is that you're just letting yourself go so you're you're supported your hands are on those legs let's do that one more

time just like that so nice long spine hands are resting on the thighs Palms are facing down right they're just kind of arms are kind of hanging between the legs let that heart fall forward tuck that chin let the head fall it's just a seated child's pose and let's roll it up okay so that's a great version and if you want to stick with that version that's great if you're with me and you're feeling okay and you want a little bit more I'm going to come to that same version of child's pose but what I'm going to do is then I'm going to take my arms off of my legs and I'm going to let myself fall a little further maybe I'm just going to hold on to my ankles or maybe your feet go to the floor right so I'm going to let you decide what feels best for you and if at any time you get dizzy getting the head below the heart then don't do that just lift your heart back into your head back up and keep your head above the heart okay so let's give it a try see what we think let's come into that first of all

that child's pose then if you want the little bit more you're going to go ahead and grab your ankles and let that heart fall a little further and then maybe your hands go down to the floor so now we're in a seated forward fold so we've moved from from Child's pose into seated forward fold we're going to let our head fall I'm kind of looking behind my chair I'm looking under my chair and back if that feels okay for you nice stretch for the back and for the upper that lower back upper back I'm

even feeling my neck stretching okay ready we're going to grab our thighs let's hold on as we come up slowly okay I want you to support yourself protect that low back and I don't want you to get dizzy okay so the very final thing we're going to do we're going to get back into whatever version you like child or forward fold then if it feels okay you're going to let go grab your elbows and we'll hang out in ragdoll now rag doll is going to give you even more stretch for the back okay so that's

kind of where you're going to feel it so let's do it again this is your version if you want to hang out in child's pose this is your version if you want to come on down into that forward fold go ahead and let the head fall if that feels okay for your body now you're going to take your hands off of your ankles or the floor you're going to grab your elbows and hang out in that ragdolls so there's the back a lot just stretching into that back we have one more breath here all right drop your

hands first now go ahead and put your hands on one on each thigh tuck the chin and roll it up into seated and take a little break how did that feel I love that so that is an inversion right so anytime we get our head below our heart is an inversion and if it makes you dizzy don't do it it's okay but it feels good to me I like it from my back and uh so anyway all right so if we're all feeling good then we're going to come up to standing and we're going to be on the right side of our chair

now this is series that is a little bit of body awareness okay so if it makes you uncomfortable to close your eyes you're going to keep your eyes open and that's going to be fine but maybe you just soften the Gaze right so instead of looking out maybe you're just soften that gaze don't let your head fall just your eyes kind of fall this bring our hands to our heart now I'm going to go ahead and close my eyes it feels okay for me but I want you to do what feels good for you pull that belly in right belly belly belly this is not balanced so if you want to hold the chair you can bring your hands to Heart we're going to rock our weight forward into the balls of our feet then we're going to bring the weight back Center then I want you to lean the weight into the heels and lift all 10 toes you're going to put all 10 toes back down on the mat we're going to lean a little bit to the right that left foot stays down though it doesn't come up off the mat bring your White Center we're going to lean the other way

bring the White Center let's bring our weight forward the heels stay down but the weight is in the balls of the feet let's bring the weight Center now bring the weight into the heels lift the five toes of your right foot starting with your pinky you're going to put them down one at a time lift the five toes of the other foot starting with your big toe you're going to put them down one at a time bring your weight forward Center Lean Back lift all ten toes and place all ten toes on the mat lean to the left

come Center lean to the right calm Center and release very good we're going to come into an extended Mountain pose but it's going to be a little different than what we're I have done in the past so we're going to bring our hands up but I want you to think like hugging a tree so instead of the arms nice and long they're going to have a little bit of Bend pull your belly in now we're going to lean forward just a little bit don't don't feel like you've got to lean too far forward

and then we're going to come up come back to goal post arms now you're going to take your left palm and you're going to bring it across to your right arm don't bring the arm to the Palm make your this hand come forward then we're going to open and then we're going to take our right hand and bring it across don't bring the left hand forward to meet it make your right hand come all the way across then we're going to lean and come Center and lean and come Center Arms up hug your tree

Lean Forward and up we go post arms one arm comes across and Center other arm comes across and Center lean and Center lean and Center what's next up hug your tree a little brain work right you remember what's next can we do that one more time without any cues we've got this ah what's next do you remember Lee yeah and release very good all right let's come to seated so we're going to move forward in our chair and take those feet a little bit wide okay now you're going to let your knees fall to the right put your hand back here on the chair behind you now if it feels okay let's let's do this again before we add on let's bring the knees up and then we're going to let those knees fall the other way so I want to give you this version first okay and it's a great version and then bring those knees up now if you want a little bit more you're going to bring the knees over then you're going to pick this knee up this leg up excuse me and place that foot on that leg so you're going to get more stretch here hold on to that chair behind you lifting up through the heart shoulders or back I know right a little bit more stretch there I feel it too one more breath okay let's take this foot off bring the knees up now we're going to let those knees fall the other way and then we're going to pick that foot

up and we're going to place it on the outside of that leg oh my God that's quite a stretch for me I don't know about you but I feel that one one more breath here okay let's take the foot off bring those knees up and sit back let's move into shavasana pose hands are going to rest lightly on those thighs we're leaning back if you want let those Palms up to the ceiling close your eyes take a deep breath in and a full breath out best version of you no feeling lasts forever if the way you feel is holding you back

change it right now you can replace futility with hope right now you can transform apathy into enthusiasm have you had a disappointing few minutes or day or month here is where the disappointment ends and a more fruitful fulfilling life begins you will always face challenges and difficult situations yet you don't ever have to let any outside conditions get you down you decide who you are how you feel where to focus your attention and energy decide in a way that uplifts your life and the lives around you the world is as it is

meet that world with the very best version of you and do the good work to bring more positive possibilities to life take a deep breath in and a full breath out drop your right ear towards your right shoulder reach up with the right hand give the head a gentle tug pressing that left hand down towards the floor release it drop your chin towards your chest reach up with the hands give the head a gentle tug release it drop your left ear towards your left shoulder reach up with the left hand give the head a gentle tug pressing that right hand down towards the floor release it look up just slightly open your mouth if you want to stretch your jaw bring your hands to your heart

DAY 22

let's get started so we're going to move forward in our chair we're going to sit up really tall crown of the head to the ceiling we're not leaning back we're going to take just a moment to focus on that mind and body and breath so let's take think about grounding our feet to the Earth and think about granting our sits bones to the chair right lift our heart lower those shoulders down out of the ears place your hands lightly on the thighs flipping the Palms up to the ceiling close your eyes and then just connect to your breath just feel the rhythm of your natural inhalation and exhalation just take your time here right so we're connecting with that breath just one more breath here bring your hands to your heart set your intentions for today's practice one more breath here bring your hands back down to your thighs and open your eyes let's go ahead and we're just going to look side to side so let's look to the right a little bit excuse me and then we're going to look Center and then we're going to look to the left and Center let's do that one more time loose looking to the right just a little stretch for the neck this morning well

it's morning for me I don't know where what time you're doing it and then we're going to go the other side I am in center and now we're going to drop our hands down by our side and we're going to shrug those shoulders up into the ears and then we're going to let them fall and we're going to shrug those shoulders up into the ears and we're going to let them fall and we're going to do that one more time shrug and just let them fall very good okay so I'm going to take my right ear

and I'm going to let it just fall towards my shoulder so a little stretch here for the neck again ah so feel your first of all just feel your natural range of motion so we're just going to hang out here for a couple of more breaths then all I want you to do is reach up with your hand and place it lightly on the head okay so we're not pulling on that we're not do you need any you know assistance we're just simply letting the weight of the hand give that a little more stretch take that hand off and bring that head

up oh my goodness that feels good to me let's go the other side so first of all just let your head go right so ear to shoulder we're just hanging out here we're feeling the stretch first now if you want a little more you're just going to take your hand and lay it lightly on the head so it's interesting to me how just the weight of the hand and a little bit of gravity really adds to that stretch all right let's take the hand off and let's lift that head up oh my that feels good to me all right

so we're going to move into our Mountain pose so we're going to bring our hands down by our side and spread those fingers nice and wide so throughout this entire pose I want you to think about lengthening through the spine crown of the head to the ceiling shoulders are down right so belly stays tight it looks like we're not doing much in this pose but it's a very active pose I'm spreading my fingers I'm stretching all right now we're going to release the fingers and we're going to come up into those goal

post arms so again I'm really pressing my arms back I'm squeezing my shoulder blades back behind me it's a very active pose lengthening up hands to the ceiling so my shoulders stay down they tend to want to come with right the minute I begin to lengthen those hands up to the ceiling but I want you to pull those shoulders down and just try to think about fingers to ceiling but shoulders are down belly is tight very active it's a little yin yang right extending and pulling one more breath and release

all right excellent work so we're going to move into some pelvic tilt so all of these beginning poses are for warm up right we kind of know that now we've done this enough so we're going to move into a little pelvic tail so this is kind of to warm up into that lower spine so we're going to take our hip tips these pointy bones here on the pelvis and we're going to rot them towards our shoulders so just kind of rounding a little bit right so you should feel that low back rounding now we're going to take these

same hip tips and we're going to rock them towards our knees there we go so now there's a little arch in the back and we're going to do that again oh yeah and the other way so it's a little bit like cat and cow right it's the same feeling if you will but it's just a little bit lower in the back okay let's add the breath we're going to inhale into our tip hip tips to shoulders and then exhale as we take the hip tips to the knees and do that a few more times inhale and exhale inhale

and exhale can we do one more inhale if you don't want to do the inhale and exhale just breathe normally right so remember you don't ever have to do that inhale and exhale with the movement of the poses and then come back to that neutral spine I want you to just breathe though you don't ever want to hold our breath okay so our next pose is a chair pose series now in chair pose the first thing

I want you to think about is we definitely want our knees to be behind our toes however I will tell you if you have your toes

too far out and try to get up out of the chair it is really hard right I mean it's almost impossible so what you want to do is make sure that you have your feet back knees are still behind the toes but you kind of want that 90 degrees down so when you press your feet and down into the feet you can lift okay so go ahead and take a moment to kind of get the position of your feet that makes sense for you okay so now we're going to bring our hands to our well actually let's start with our hands on our thighs so I like

to start here give yourself a little support and then we'll add on hands to heart so we're going to inhale to prepare and then as we exhale I want you to press your hands into your thighs we're going to act like we're getting out of the chair but we're not going to get out of the chair so you've got to use your quadriceps and your belly inhale to prepare exhale just act like you're going to lift your hips up but don't and we're breathing here we're not holding our breath and then we're going

to release that do you feel that a lot of work in those quads and abdominals it's almost like easier to just lift up but we're not going to yet and how to prepare ready exhale press try to lift those hips up but don't right they're just barely barely barely coming up off the chair we have one more breath and release it we're gonna do that one more time just like that inhale exhale press then just breathe your natural breath don't hold it one more breath and release okay so we're gonna do that same thing with our

hands at heart all right we're not lifting up we're just gonna act like we're gonna get out of the chair but we don't we really feel your abdominals working and your quadriceps working all right hands to Heart inhale to prepare exhale act like you're gonna get up and down oh yeah one more breath and down we go let's do that again inhale exhale hold and breathe and release one more time inhale exhale press up one more breath and release okay take just a little break here so now we're actually going to go ahead

and come up out of that chair so I'm going to start with hands at heart but I will tell you if you want to start with hands and thighs that's fine give yourself that little extra support it's okay all right inhale to prepare exhale now let's come all the way up so if you'll notice I'm going to turn to the side so you can see me just a little bit see how my knees are behind my toes my hips are back okay so here I am in a chair pose and my heart is lifted here's what I will see sometimes in my in-person classes here I am in my chair pose well what that does is it disconnects the quadriceps and the abdominals right you're just kind of resting here that's not the pose here's the pose right heart is lifted hips are back knees are behind toes hands are at heart all right go ahead and have a seat okay let's do that again inhale to prepare exhale lift up into your chair pose so my abdominals are really engaged here my quadriceps are working hard my heart is lifted I'm not letting myself

collapse down one more breath have a c so one more thing I want you to think about before we add this last piece on when you come back to seated there's something that's called just awareness of you of your vicinity and what's going on around you right so I guarantee you nobody has come and moved to that chair so you don't have to turn and look and sit we want to work on a little spatial awareness here a little spatial awareness so as you come up let's everybody come back up hands at heart now

that chair's there you've got some spatial awareness of what's going on around you and you're going to sit back down okay it's really good for the brain to do that let's do that one more time inhale to prepare exhale up we go now the fur another add-on is extending the arms out only if it feels good for you this is this now do you feel your back engaging right so extending those arms out adds a little back work bring your hands to heart and have a seat okay the final add-on in how to prepare exhale up we go

let's extend those arms now we're going to come to standing ha inhale to prepare exhale chair pose bring your hands to heart and have a seat inhale exhale chair pose extend your arms inhale to prepare exhale stand up ah inhale down we go hands to Heart have a seat can we do one more I know one more here we go press it up extend those arms up we go okay are we ready and have a seed how did that feel I know right a lot of work that but it's a lot of work okay so we're gonna do a little stretch now this one should feel really

good we're going to take our right knee and we're going to open it up nice and wide here alright so this feels like a quite a stretch on those inner thighs just to start with so the thing I want you to focus in on is this knee that's facing me I guarantee you it's going to want to fold in but I don't want you to let it okay so I want you to really keep this knee open now if it just is just not going to stay open then I'd rather you heel toe your foot in just a little bit I'd rather you keep that alignment of hip knee ankle and toes and do the twist versus be here and let the knee fall out does that make sense all right I was talking but I wanted you to feel the stretch on that inner thigh while I was talking we're going to bring this left arm out and bring it all you know open up now you're going to bring that arm all the way across your body and you're going to grab your chair I want you to look lengthen nice and long through the spine and I want you to turn and look over the back of your chair now everybody turn and look at

your knee what's happening is it folding then if it's folding in you can either make sure it's not or you can bring that foot in a little bit right oh my goodness go ahead and look back over the back of your chair again feel that stretch and open open that arm and then let's do that again ready let's bring that arm across the body lift don't forget the lifting through the crown of the head and then twist that's super important we have one more breath release bring that knee forward so the other thing

that's really important in any twist or stretch or whatever if we're going to move that spine in any direction we want it long before we start okay so we always lift crown of the head to the ceiling before we turn all right let's do the other side here we go open it up feeling that stretch first ah bring your right arm open it up first and then bring it all the way across the body grab the chair what do we do next lift the spine crown of the head to the ceiling turn look over the back of your chair make sure that right knee is open

don't let it fold in one more breath let's release that and we're going to do it one more time we got this all the way across the body grab the chair lift and twist we just have one more breath open up and release okay excellent work so the next pose is star pose from a seated position so we're going to do a little heel toe heel toe all right now what I'd like for you to do is hold the chair pull that belly in and I just want you to lengthen the legs long and bring them in okay we're just kind

of getting used to this movement extend and bend okay you feeling that extend and bend let's do that one more time before we add on extend and bend okay so now we're going to do the same thing but we're going to add our arms so our arms are going to come up into like a V okay and then down okay can we do both at the same time inhale to prepare exhale up inhale down does that feel okay let's do that again up and down two more up there's our star and down one more up and down Okay so let's bring our feet back together good work so now the next thing it doesn't seem like it's going to be that much of a difference but I think you'll see the difference so instead of starting with our legs out we're going to start with our legs together all right so now they have to move into that full extension and bend in abdominals okay so we're going to just go for it we're not gonna if you want to grab that chair remember that's always an option but if you're with me we're going to bring our hands to Heart

inhale to prepare ready exhale up inhale down exhale up inhale now you feeling it exhale up inhale down let's do three more up and down into star pose up and down let's do one more belly tight don't lean back and down and release all right mine is mine's my my Bloods are pumping a little bit all right very very good so the next series is going to be a little flow we're going to start in a warrior two and we're going to move into a reverse Warrior and the side angle pose now what we're the atoms here isn't

going to be adding on more poses is going to be adding on the position of our legs and you'll see how we continue to build into a little deeper stretch and a little deeper stretch and remember you don't have to add on right so if you get into that first position and then you try to go into the next one where we're you know a little deeper stretch you're like I don't think so then just go right back to that previous version okay so it's it's fine that's why I do it this way so I give everybody the

opportunity to be super successful in all of these series all right so we're going to start in our Warrior Two And what I want you to do is just take your right knee and open it so we did this one a minute ago so we kind of know how this feels right now you're going to kind of turn your torso to face me and you're going to bring those arms up so this is our Warrior Two so I want you to think about having your arms parallel to the mat right so I'll see in my classes I'll have this or I'll

have that right extend the arms as long as you can belly is tight all right now we're going to flip this right palm is is considered our front Palm the right palm is going to flip up and then we're going to reverse our Warrior so here's the thing if you want to hold the chair it's okay if you think it's all right for you you're going to leave that hand down and just let it slide down towards the floor so that's going to work that side waist a little bit more you might get a little more

stretch too but it's your choice right holding the chair is always an option all right let's come back to that Warrior Two now we're going to take that right arm we're going to flip the Palm to the ceiling and we're going to put that arm right on that thigh and we're going to lift up here's our side angle pose now we might extend that side angle here in a minute bringing this arm over but for now I want you to leave it out at a diagonal so I've got shoulder shoulder wrist right in alignment do you feel

that hard opening you this this side is working right it's working to keep that openness happening so if you're feeling like you're kind of collapsing in I want you to really make it to where you're opening up into that chest okay are we ready inhale exhale back to that Warrior Two now squeeze the muscles against the bones in the arm so what does that mean if I came over and I tried to pull your arm down I couldn't right so you're squeezing activating that upper body we have one more breath let's release that okay

let's bring that foot in now we're going to go to the other side all right before we add on so here we go let's bring that knee open extend Warrior Two look over your left fingertips that's our front hand Now flip that Palm to the ceiling reverse your Warrior if you can look up towards the ceiling do so if you can bring that hand past the midline of the body do so belly stays tight let's come back to that Warrior Two and we're going to move into our side angle pose right looking out for me works best you can look up but I

thought I personally at least like looking out we have one more breath let's press back up into Warrior Two and release and bring that knee in okay so now we're going to move through that a little bit faster with a little bit of additional legs okay so I'm just going to let you decide if you want to stay in this position with your legs that's fine if you want the next version I'm going to take my right knee and it's going to be a heel toe and a heel toe so it's at a diagonal right it's not 90 degrees

it's at that diagonal probably like a 40 45 degrees all right the opposite leg extends out so you see what's happening there I've gotten a lot more stretch happening on this extended leg now I'm up on the side of that foot so if you point your toe and extend now your quadricep is working that's there's nothing wrong with that but really what this pose is is uh intended to Accent or activate I should say the inner and outer thigh right so if this particular series we're working on that inner outer thigh and so in

order to get that area engaged I bend my foot I flex my foot and I'm up on the edge okay so I feel you feel it you should feel it already right here okay let's bring those arms up to that Warrior Two we're going to move right through this we're not going to stop all right look over those right fingertips flip that Palm up to the ceiling reverse your Warrior up and back come back to that Warrior Two and we're going to put that arm on that leg flip the Palm up into that side angle pose you're going to flip back up into that

Warrior Two front Palm up and back back to Warrior Two straight to side angle pose one more time Warrior Two reverse Warrior Warrior Two to side angle back to Warrior Two and release ah feel okay ready for the other side here we go heel toe heel toe extend that right leg out make sure you're on the side of the foot bring those arms up to that Warrior too shoulders your down belly is tight look over those left fingertips flip that Palm to the ceiling reverse the warrior up and back we're going to come back to that Warrior

Two into our side angle pose press into that Warrior Two flip that Palm up and back back to your Warrior Two into side angle pose beautiful Series right back to that Warrior Two you guys are doing great flip that Palm up and back a little movement here and back to Warrior Two back to side angle one more breath bring your hands down bring that leg in and take a break work all right okay so we're going to move into gate pose so what I want you to do is move towards the right side of your chair okay so I caught I've got a

hair here that's bugging me there we go sorry so I moved to the right side of my chair you're going to hold on to that chair and you're going to extend that left leg I mean right like sorry rightly send that right leg out so again I'm up on the edge of that foot okay oh yeah okay so now what I'm going to do is I'm going to lift my arm up and I'm going to lean over as I close my gate you feel that oh yeah that's working that sideways now I'm going to bring that hand back to the chair

I'm going to extend the opposite arm up and lean so now I'm opening my gate I'm still feeling that sideways stretching right and down we go now if you want you can have that right arm so the left arm extends up the right arm can just slide down that leg if that feels okay and then up we go opposite arm extends do you feeling that a little stretch there for that so inner outer thigh is getting it and now we're getting into that side waist and up we go let's do that one more time well when I say one more time we've got

two sides right so it's really kind of two times opposite arm extends and we lean oh that feels good to me and up we go and release okay take a moment here on that chair we got to do the other side so we're doing a little more moving today aren't we right so we're not really holding our poses as long we're moving through them it's just different it's all good uh both versions are excellent let's extend that leg okay so take a moment here make sure you feel like you're stable on that chair

we've got this leg extended we're up on the side of that foot okay all right so we're going to take our right hand we're going to extend it up left hand is on that leg and we're going to lean and close our gate they were going to come up erase that hand on the mat extend the other hand and open our gate and then up we go extend and Link hand to the chair extend and lean we have one more we got this feeling that movement that flow ah last one oh that feels so good and up we got very very good go ahead and come to seated for just a

moment here all right let's come to standing beside our chair now we're going to move into a standing Sun salutation B and what the B is is the chair pose series okay so we're going to move pretty fluidly through the beginning of our sun salutation focusing a little bit more into that chair pose okay so I like to move a little bit forward in my chair because we're going to be moving those arms right for that Swan Dive and if you're if you're a little bit too far back you might hit the back of the chair

so just think about that bring your hands to Heart okay reverse one dive up to Mountain pose and then bring your hands to heart now if you can follow your hands yeah with your gaze that's great if not don't worry about it just look forward inhale up we go exhale we're going to Swan Dive forward belly button to spine forward salute airplane arm so I'm stretching my fingers back my head is forward I'm stretching through and I'm going to bring my hands to Heart let's do that one more time and we'll move

away from my chair just a little bit and reversalon dive up to Mountain pose bring your hands to Heart add the breath if you want it inhale up exhale die forward okay now we're going to put our hands on our thighs and give ourselves a little support for our first forward fold oh yeah letting that heart begin to fall forward and our hands are on my thighs for some support my head is staying above my heart I'm going to bend my knees tuck my chin and roll it up into a standing position hands to Heart let's

do that again reverse lung die up inhale here exhale hands to Heart up we go on that inhale if you want to add that breath dive It Forward High forward salute airplane arms stretch it out hands on thighs forward fold bend the knees roll it up into a standing position okay so now I'm going to add one thing in here so instead of having the hands on the thighs for support I'm going to go ahead and just have my hands out and then let's reverse one dive up that doesn't work for your back you're going to stay here and bend

the knees and roll up which is a fine version okay but I'm going to add in a little bit of back work okay here we go big circle up Mountain pose bring your hands to Heart let's come back to Mountain belly button to spine diving forward forward salute airplane arms we're going to stretch that out let's place our hands on our thighs for a supported forward fold to start with okay now if you feel okay and your back is good pull that belly button in you're going to release the hands and then reverse Swan Dive all the way back up to

Mountain pose and bring your hands to Heart let's do that just like that one more time up we go dive It Forward ha forward salute airplane arm stretch supported forward fold to start with hands off of those thighs reverse one die back up we go to Mountain pose bring your hands to your heart we're going to add on from here are we ready up we go diving forward belly button to spine forward salute airplane arms supported forward fold bend your knees shoot your hips back bring your hands to Heart and come into chair pose

oh yeah extend those arms out now we're going to come into a forward fold if you want to just forward fold hands towards the floor go for it if you want to put your hands on thighs that's fine reverse Swan dog all the way back up to Mountain pose bring your hands to Heart how are you feeling that makes you dizzy don't do it right keep your hand head above your heart dive it forward we got this forward-solute airplane arms ready supported forward fold bend the knee shoot the hips back bring the hands to heart for chair pose extend

those arms if you wish there's the back you feel it hands to heart heart to thighs hands to the mat reverse Swan Dive up we go we got one more that's it one more hands to Heart feeling okay up we go I know right moving we're flowing today halfway lift well forward salute airplane arms supported forward fold bend the knees hands to Heart chair pose extend the arms out hands to Heart to thighs hands to the mat straighten those legs reverse Swan Dive all the way back up Mountain pose and bring your hands to

your heart excellent work that was a great flow excellent okay so the next one we're going to do we're going to stand here we've got our chair right here by us we're going to move into some Eagle legs with a warrior three so I want you to put the weight in the leg next to the chair lift the other knee up to tabletop okay so first of all bring your right hand to to your heart pull that belly in super tight see if you can let go of that chair and bring the other hand up there's a little balance work right

yellow okay so now the leg that's in the air I'm gonna push it through to a warrior three with prayer hands so do you see how I'm still lifting my heart right I'm not letting my heart fall down see I needed to grab the chair just for a moment that's fine I'll let go now okay let's do that again bring that knee up and then press that foot back how is that working for you I know belly right use those abdominals pelvic floor muscles lift find a spot that's not moving focus in on that bring that knee

up let's do that one more time push that foot back now if you want one final add-on we're going to go to airplane arms so instead of hands to prayer three two one nice and slow bring that knee up squeeze it put that foot on the floor okay let's go to the other side so it's a little moving balance a little dynamic balance right so we're going to put the weight into the leg next to the chair we're going to bring that opposite knee up eagle leg table top leg belly tight let's bring this left hand to the heart to start

with now if you think you can you're going to bring the other hand up working that balance okay are we ready we're gonna push that foot through into that Warrior three do you notice how kind of my upper body doesn't really move much does it I want you to keep that heart lifted we're not letting that heart fall forward okay let's bring that knee up ready push it through I know I know it's challenging it's challenging for me too belly tight and up we go so this side could be more willing though than the

other right super common to have one side more than the other let's push that through okay we ready for those airplane arms we have one more breath come up bring that knee up into the chest and put that foot down mindfully remember we always want to get out of our balance poses mindfully such good work you guys let's go ahead and come back to see it excellent excellent excellent okay we're going to take our right knee and we're going to open it and let our left knee fall down for that Crescent

lunge push that foot back ah lift that heart let's bring the arms to goal post and squeeze our shoulder blades back behind you it's just a little extra stretch here let's release that and we're going to do that one more time ready oh that feels good let's release that and face forward okay can we do the other side now so we're going to take that other knee and open it wide this knee is going to fall straight down towards the floor push that foot back lift your heart so start here so relaxing through this glute feeling

the stretch on this front side of that leg let's come to goal post arms and squeeze I'm shoulder Bliss behind us looking up a little bit if that feels okay let's release it I'm going to do that one more time and release go ahead and face forward we're going to move into shavasana pose so you can lean back on the chair hands are going to rest lightly on the thighs flip the Palms up to the ceiling take a deep breath in and as you exhale close your eyes take another deep breath in and a full breath out

making a difference life in all its forms has made a difference long before you were around to see it vast stretches of hard unyielding volcanic rock were transformed into soft fertile soil by the power of life the oxygen that sustains you in every moment is constantly replenished by life itself much of the value in your world comes from the reality that life in its very essence makes a difference not only can you make a difference you can choose what difference to make every day you make that choice and every

day it matters you can positively affect the course of your own life and the lives around you it is magnificent opportunity and a great responsibility what you think what you choose what you do it all makes a difference far beyond what anyone can imagine so it's best to make your choices based on love wisdom gratitude respect and generosity all the time you can make a difference you do make a difference what positive and uplifting difference will you make right now take a deep breath in and a full breath out

drop your right ear towards your right shoulder reach up with the right hand give the head a gentle tug as the left hand presses down towards the floor release it drop your chin towards your chest reach up with your hands give the head a gentle tongue release it drop your left ear towards your left shoulder reach up with the left hand give the head a gentle tug pressing that right hand down towards the floor release it look up just slightly open your mouth if you want to stretch your jaw bring your hands to your heart

DAY 23

we're going to sit up tall in our chair we're not leaning back we're going to focus in on that mind and body and breath take both of your feet ground them to the Earth they're equally weighted on that floor the sits bones are grounded to the chair you're not leaning one way or the other heart is lifted shoulders are down out of the ears hands are lightly on the thighs let's flip those Palms up towards the ceiling we're gonna close our eyes and just feel your natural inhalation and exhalation focusing on your heart center elongate that breath inhale and looply exhale a little more completely

do that again inhale and exhale and breathe normally bring your hands to your heart set your intentions for today's practice one more breath here bring your hands back down to your thighs and open your eyes we're gonna shrug our shoulders up into our ears and then we're just gonna let them fall and then we're gonna do that again just shrug those shoulders up and let them fall one more time and just let them fall doesn't work we're going to draw that right ear to that right shoulder we're

going to reach up with the right hand just lay it lightly on the head extend that opposite arm out flexing through the wrist pushing through the palm of the hand so you're almost getting a little more stretch because of the arm extension I'm not pulling on this right if the head hand is just resting on that head from Center we're going to do the other side all right let's do it let's draw that ear to the shoulder first and you're just going to reach up with the hand just lightly place it there on the head and the

opposite arm extends pushing through the palm alright let's all come back Center and release that all right very good I'm going to move my head just a little bit does that feel okay good moving into Mountain pose another warm-up pose extending those arms out spreading those fingers come to go post arms squeezing the shoulder blades back behind you and fingertips to the ceiling High shoulders or down belly is tight one more breath here bring the hands down we're going to do that again here we go bring those arms out spreading

those fingers nice and wide for a stretch come to those goal post arms really squeeze your shoulder blades back behind you now taking those fingertips to the ceiling shoulders are down trying to touch the ceiling with your fingertips one more breath and bring those hands down and take just a little break all right very good so I'm going to move a little forward in my chair we're going to do some shoulder dips so let's do a heel toe heel toe so my knees are nice and wide I've got an alignment of hips

to knees to ankles to toes okay so all in alignment alright so my hands are just going to rest right here on my thighs and I'm going to let my right shoulder just dip right between my legs so there's the side waist working stretching should feel good then we're going to bring that shoulder up and then we're going to let the other shoulder fall down right between those legs so I'm feeling a little bit of inner thigh stretching and working belly is tight here and let's come up okay so you're going to do that again

just letting that shoulder dip down feeling the stretch side waist is working belly is tight up we go let's do the other side shoulder dips here and we're gonna do that one more time on each side I know it just feels good lift and let's do the other side and lift okay we're gonna bring those feet in together now excellent so I'm going to bring my right knee up and into my chest so I have a nice long spine crown of the head to the ceiling now you're going to round just like we maybe like a cat's pose and

you're gonna maybe drop your knee your nose to your knee and then lift it up so it's a little rounding of the spine upper back is rounding as I come down and my knee my nose comes to my knee and then lift up we're gonna do that one more time round it down maybe the nose maybe it's the forehead right and then up we go and put that foot down okay let's do the other side so I'm going to hug my knee up into my chest to begin with now I will tell you if this bothers your knee maybe you hold back

behind your thigh which is fine right absolutely fine okay we ready we're going to drop our nose towards our knee doesn't have to touch don't worry I just want you to think about rounding and then lift it up and let's do that again round and down think about nose to knee or forehead to knee doesn't matter and then lift it up we're going to do that one more time round it down and lift it up and place that foot on the floor okay really good so now this next one is uh that one was a little bit

more for the upper back and the and rounding right in the shoulders this one is going to be more for the leg so we're going to lift holding under that thigh we're going to lift that knee up so same idea here just like we did a minute ago now what

I want you to do is flex and then I want you to push extending the leg then we're going to bend that knee and we're going to put that foot on the floor let's do it again same side ex up Flex extend bend the knee and put the foot on the floor again bring the knee up Flex extend

bring the knee in and foot on the floor now we're going to go to the other side okay so here we go we're going to bring that knee up and in first flex the foot now extend the leg bend the knee and put the foot on the floor are you keeping your abdominals tight are you keeping that nice long spine so we don't want to lean back and we don't want to slouch right and foot down let's do that again bring it in Crown of the head to the ceiling extend Bend and foot to the floor okay so we're going to do that exact same

thing again but we're not going to hold our left hook all right so we're just going to have our hands resting on our thighs ready lift Flex extend Bend foot to the floor switch sides lift flex extend Bend foot to the floor switch sides lift flex extend Bend foot to the floor switch sides lift flex extend up we go all right the little final add on here we go lift flex extend hold for three two one Bend put the foot on the floor other side lift flex extend hold four three two one Bend put the foot on the floor last

time on each side lift flex extend hold for three two one Bend put the foot on the floor don't lean back Flex extend crown of the head to the ceiling two one Bend and put that foot on the floor excellent work you guys so so good I'm gonna be back just a little bit on my chair so that I feel a little more stable now we're going to bring our arms our forearms are parallel in front of the body just a light fist okay so I'm not just a super light fist here okay so I'm going to bring that arm out

and then I'm going to bring It Center and then the other side out and Center let's do that again out and center and out and Center okay so bring those arms down now we're going to do the legs okay so let's hold that chair we're going to bring that leg open and close and open and close again open close open and close okay so now we're going to put those two things together so your abdominals have got to stay engaged your inner and outer thighs are going to be working pretty hard so there's quite a

bit going on with the lower body okay so we're going to come up to those parallel arms before we start I suggest you move a little bit forward in your chair it's going to make the leg movement a little more fluid for you so don't be too far back in that chair okay so here we go four arms are parallel to the front of the body are we ready we're going to move that arm and the leg at the same time let's start on the right side here we go open and close switch sides open and close switch sides open

close open close again open close last one last Side open and close and release how did that feel little inner outer thigh work right so our next series is a crescent lunge variation so we've done Chris if you've been with me through this series we've done Crescent lunge right that's one of our kind of staple go-to's especially to stretch the front side of the leg well this is going to be a little different in the sense that we're going to be doing some stuff of the upper body that we haven't done before so we're going to

take our right knee and we're going to open it first right then we're going to take that left knee and we're going to let it fall down towards the floor okay does that make sense that feeling okay all right so now we're going to take this hand of the knee that's extending we're going to bring it right here to our shoulder then I want you to extend like this shoulder is down towards that leg and then we're going to come up and let's do that again and let's do that one more time are you

feeling a little extra stretch there and that side waist is working and up okay now let's release that knee take a little break we're going to do the other side so we're going to bring that hand let's go ahead and extend this leg back again relaxing into this glute the other hand is here and then we're going to come down elbow towards the seat of the chair and up so feeling the side waist working pretty hard here we're squeezing the side of that waist and then up and let's do it one more

time and then up then let's relax that leg we just have one little add-on okay one final thing so we're going to extend back now this arm instead of on the shoulder and squeezing we're going to go the other way so I'm going to bring it across the body you see what I'm doing there and then I'm going to bring it back and then I'm going to bring it across the body and then I'm going to bring it back let's do one more and back hands to the chair and release okay did that feel okay I know right it's a

little different it's kind of nice because we're we're doing a little bit more into the sideways for those oblique muscles right those sideways muscles okay it's we got this we're going to do the other side now it's not nearly as complicated as it seems right so let's take that knee open it opposite knee falls down and remember I don't think I said this on the other side but if you want that knee just to go straight down towards the floor that's fine that right that version is fine I'm going to go ahead

and push mine back a little bit because I have that availability in the quadricep and the hip flexor feels like a good stretch for me all right so here we go we're going to take out this outside hand we're going to place it right here on that shoulder now you can hold the chair or if you want to make your muscles your oblique muscles work harder don't hold the chair just place this hand here on the thigh and we're going to squeeze that side waist so it's kind of like right here this area I'm

squeezing and then let's come up let's do that again squeeze and come up do it two more times squeeze and up one more time squeeze come up let's release that now we're going to do the other side okay so now this hand comes to this shoulder extend that leg back if that's what you're doing engage this leg in whatever way you're engaging it and then we're going to squeeze and release let's do that again and release we've got two more we have one more all right come up relax this leg for

just a moment final version this outside arm is going to come across the body all right so let's extend that leg out bring this arm up and across the body so now we're adding the back so it's sideways and back and then come Center let's do that again and come Center a little crescent lunge variation we have one more I'm feeling a lot of muscles in my lower body I don't know about you and upper this feels a lot like a full body stretch here and since here we go and release how did that feel

right I mean you don't think again you don't think that we're doing too much there until we get it all added in together and boy it's a full body work and stretch really really good so the next thing we're going to do is this is some core work so we're going to act like we're rowing a boat all right so we're going to bring we got our paddle here right and we're going to bring it to this side again sideways muscles and abdominals are working and then we're going to bring these arms to

the other side you see if I'm kind of twisting there my knees are staying forward let's do that again rowing that boat and up and rolling on the other side and up again row and up row and up let's do that one more time row and up last time last side row and up and release okay so now the add-on is we're going to lift our knee so if the if we're rowing on the right we're going to lift our right knee okay so here we go let's see how that feels make sure you're stable on the chair we're going to row and up now I'm going to the left side so my left leg is lifting and up and roll and up row and again lifting that knee putting it down other side let's do it one more time on each side we have one more add-on and let's release that okay so the final add-on is we're doing both arms at the same time and lifting both legs at the same time so really working the abdominals here so instead of going side to side we're going to stay in the center let's just do our arms first kind of see what I'm doing here getting the feeling of it okay now pull your belly in super tight here we go we're going to lift legs and row lift and down lift and down lift and down one more lift and down excellent excellent excellent okay so the next series is called liftoff we're going to come from seated and we're going to stand up and then we're going to sit down and we're going to stand up and we're going to sit down so it's just a up and down motion you want your feet to be back a little bit you want your knees to be behind your toes

but you're going to want those feet back just a little bit think about chair pose right if you were with me I think it was yesterday maybe day before yesterday that we did that chair pose okay so we're gonna start hands on thighs inhale exhale press it up and see it sit down press it up and sit down press it up and sit down press it up I know right belly tight sit down press it up sit down two more press it up sit down last one press it up sit down now take a little break get your heart rate up a little bit

okay so the next thing we're going to do is we're going to cross our arms at our chest so instead of using our arms to help us press up now we've got to use our legs only and abdominals okay so we're going to cross those arms remember this is an add-on you don't ever have to add on you keep doing this version are we ready in how to prepare exhale press it up and sit down there's ten president and nine are we ready president there's eight oh yeah press it up there's seven whoa press it up there's six

and five four three two now listen stay standing yay we did it that was excellent I call those liftoff I don't know that's a there's not really a name for us specifically but that's kind of what I call it all right excellent work we're going to come behind our chair and we're going to do horse pose okay so with some calf raises so I'm gonna do a heel toe heel toe so my feet are at a diagonal my knees are in alignment with those toes hold that chair pull that belly in and then I want you to

shoot your hips back and come into your goddess legs okay getting ready for horse pose hold that chair okay we're going to lift our right heel up off the floor and then we're going to put that heel down we're going to lift our left heel up off the floor and down lift up and down lift up and down again up and down up and down now let's lift one heel then the other heel hold and breathe so both heels are off the floor belly is tight we're holding on to that chair one more breath bring those heels down straighten

the legs and bring the feet in and take a break okay so checking in how did that feel right so we're gonna add on so the first add-on is we're not going to hold the chair so we are going to start into a little bit of balance work but you've got the chair right there right so let's go ahead get into our heel toe heel toe all right bend your knees shoot your hips back belly tight heart stays lifted make sure your knees are behind your toes right okay so now see if it feels okay for you to let go of the chair and bring those

arms up to gopost Arms now we're going to lift one heel and we're going to put it down and lift the other heel and put it down we'll lift and down and lift and down one more lift and down lived and down now see if it feels okay you're going to lift both heels up off the floor belly tight three two one grab the chair straighten the legs feet ah how did that feel really good yeah yeah okay so we're just gonna do one final version and and just a little different arm placement okay so let's do

it heel toe heel toe right everything's in alignment bend your knees shoot your hips back hold that chair okay so now instead of arms at goal posts we're going to bring our arms up so kind of think like you're in airport security right in that stupid machine where you've got to do your arms up so just kind of think about that all right belly is tight here we go lift and lower other side heel up and lower switch lift and lower belly tight lift and lower shoulders down lift and lower lift and lower listen lift and lift so

here we are balancing very tight and three two one grab the chair put the feet down straighten the legs he'll toe the feet back together all right very very good okay so we're gonna do a downward facing dog this is a little variation of if you've been with me throughout the series we've done downward dog before this is going to be just a little different so you're going to stay behind your chair I'm going to turn my chair so you can see me a little bit better what I'm doing okay so I'm going to take a step back

my hands are going to be on the seat of the chair okay so I want those arms to be very long in fact I'm going to step back just a little bit more so you really want those arms to be very very long now you're going to begin to let your heart fall forward so you should be feeling a nice stretch through the vertebrae right so super long into that vertebrae now what I'm going to do is I'm going to bring my head forward so my elbows bend a little bit I'm bringing my arms I'm sorry my head forward now you're going

to bring your hips back press back you see what I'm doing there it's almost like an accordion right stretching now I'm going to bring my upper body forward again Bend those arms so I'm squeezing forward now push back oh yeah let's do that two more times come in Center and then push back you should feel a stretch in that back oh my gosh that feels good to me let's do that one more time come Center now push back feel that stretch in that spine for three two one bend the knees and roll it up

into a standing position didn't that feel good nice little stretch there for that back okay I want to do that one more time and add a little bit of breath so if it doesn't work for your body right you don't like the breathing you know the the yoga breath if you will dish breed normally but let's see if we can do that one more time now you know why we want to be so far along right so that man that feels good in that spine let's come forward so we've got the hands on that chair we're

supporting that body right I'm going to bring my feet back just a little bit more okay are we ready we're going to inhale as we come forward exhale back inhale forward exhale back inhale forward exhale back last one inhale forward exhale back Bend those knees and roll it up into seated into into standing okay so now we're going to do a quadruped and again this is a little variation of a traditional quadruped I like it a lot okay so what we're going to do is we're going to have our hands on our on the back of our chair right so

I'm stepping back just a little bit now what I'm going to do is hinge forward but I'm not as far back as I was for our for our down dog I'm going to take this left hand and I'm going to extend it out and then I'll take my right foot and I'm going to extend it so you don't want to do the same side doesn't matter which but you want to be opposite so my left arm is out and my right foot is back either is fine but you want it to be the other opposite we have one more breath let's bring that

hand back down and bring that foot forward we're going to do the other side so extending one arm out that foot is behind you standing leg is straight one more breath and come Center okay that's a really good version and if you like that version excellent so the next version we're going to step back just a little bit further okay I'm going to hinge forward now my left forearm is going to rest on that chair okay my right foot is going to come back I'm going to bend my front knee a little bit

so you've got this now pull that belly in super tight lift that right foot up off the floor Flex put the toe down lift the right foot up off the floor Flex put the toe down lift Flex put the toe down one more lift Flex put the toe down bring that foot forward going straight to the other side extend that right arm forearm is going to rest on the chair push the left foot back get your balance here belly tight we're going to lift that leg up we're going to flex the foot we're going to put the toes on the floor lift the leg up Flex the foot put the toes on the floor lift the leg up Flex the foot put the toes on the floor last one lift Flex come down bring that foot forward and roll it up so it's just a little different isn't it really really good okay let's come to seated okay so we're going to do our Crescent lunge one more time I know you're like okay well we've done a lot of Crescent lunch today but let's go ahead and we're going to open up that right knee and we're gonna let that left knee fall down

towards the floor push that leg back so just a nice supported Crescent lunge here focusing on the leg not the side like we did before okay release and let's do that one more time and face forward extend that same leg out in front of you extending nice and long through the spine pyramid pose remember looking out not down keep the back flat keep this leg straight all right let's tuck our chin and roll up and we'll do one more inhale extend exhale down we go and then just breathe naturally and we go okay let's do the other side

open let this knee fall down towards the floor pushing the foot back if that feels okay for you back of the kneecap towards the ceiling feel the stretch here heart stays lifted hold and breathe and release it and let's do that one more time up we go and release pyramid pose same leg extend it out in front of you lengthen through the spine let the heart fall forward and roll it up let's do that one more time nice and long spine exhale as you come forward keeping the back flat keeping the legs straight and up we go

very very good let's move into shavasana pose hence we're going to rest lightly on the thighs flip the Palms up to the ceiling take a deep breath in as you exhale close those eyes a job well done it's a great feeling when you know you've done something well think of what you could do today to give yourself that feeling when you make a difference it makes a difference for you suddenly you're more enthusiastic more keenly aware of life's best possibilities a job well done improves your outlook on life and raises your confidence level it enables you to connect with your skills capabilities and resourcefulness is there any task you've neglected that you could focus on today is there anything you've been doing half-heartedly that you could give more diligence and attention to be all too easy to grow cynical and disappointed with life yet whenever you choose you can create a powerful reminder of Life at its best give yourself and your world the benefit of a job well done discover all over again how positive and effective you can

be take a deep breath in and a full breath out drop your right ear towards your right shoulder reach up with the right hand give the head a gentle tug as you press that left hand down towards the floor release it drop your chin towards your chest reach up with your hands give the head a gentle tug release it drop your left ear towards your left shoulder reach up with the left hand give the head a gentle tug pressing that right hand down towards the floor release it look up just slightly open your mouth if you want to stretch your jaw bring your hands to your heart

DAY 24

we're going to start by sitting up nice and tall in our chair and moving forward so we're not leaning back we're going to take both feet we're going to place them on the floor feel like they're equally weighted as we ground them to that floor and the same thing with our sits bones we're grounding them to the chair let's lift our heart lower our shoulders down out of the ears place the hands lightly on the thighs flip the Palms up to the ceiling close the eyes and just breathe your natural breath I'm going to move that breath down into the diaphragm so as you inhale the belly

extends and we're filling the lungs from the bottom up and then as you exhale actively pulling the belly button in towards the spine pushing the air up and out of the lungs do that a couple of times and then breathe normally we're going to continue with our diaphragmatic breath we'll inhale to four counts exhale to five something like this inhale two three four exhale two three four five inhale two three four exhale two three four five and breathe normally bring your hands to your heart set your intentions for today's practice

focusing in on what you want to accomplish one more breath bring your hands down to your thighs and open your eyes we're going to roll our shoulders so it's a forward up back and down let's do that again forward up back and down and then let's reverse it back up forward and down again back up forward and down very very good okay so we're gonna grab the back of our chair all right so keep those shoulders down out of the ears but squeeze your shoulder blades back behind you now let's drop that right ear to that

right shoulder um drop your chin towards your chest feel that stretch maintain that squeeze behind you let's let the opposite ear fall down now go ahead and drop your chin towards your chest you're going to release the back of the chair and you're going to bring your hands up to the head just lay them lightly on the back of the head and let the elbows fall towards the mat so I'm not pulling on my head I'm just letting the weight of my hands and the gravity give it a little extra stretch let's release that and we're going to do

that again grab the back of your chair lift up through the heart scrap squeeze the shoulder blades back behind you let's drop that left ear first and Chin to chest drop right ear to right shoulder let's release the chair drop the chin towards the chest reach up with the hands let the hands rest lightly on the back of the head elbows down towards the floor and release all right excellent so we're going to move into our Mountain pose with just a little bit of an add-on here so let's come down we know this one well

now belly tight shoulders are down spread those fingers go post arms squeeze fingertips to the ceiling okay we're going to bring that right hand down towards the chair we're going to lengthen through that left side and then we're going to lean our Mountain now we're going to take that hand that's in the air and we're going to link and press it up towards the ceiling and turn and look up and then we're going to bring that arm across the body again for a leaning Mountain pose take the hand up to the ceiling turn and

look up it's just a little twist and then we're going to bring that leaning Mountain one more time fingers up to the ceiling bring that hand down and release it okay let's do mountain pose again we're going to go to the other side GoPro storm squeeze fingertips to the ceiling left hand to the chair right hand extends lean your Mountain take that hand to the ceiling turn and look up let's leaner Mountain hands to the ceiling turn and look up one more lean that mountain hand up look up and release all right really good so

we're going to move into a cat and a cow pose so we're going to bring our hands to our heart I want you to lift up through the spine open that throat up all right now we're going to start in cow pose we're going to grab the back of our chair lift up through the heart squeeze the shoulder blades back behind you and then we're going to move to cat's pose hands are going to come to the thighs elbows wide pull that belly button in towards the spine tuck the chin looking down at your lap take the hands to the back of the chair

lift up into your cow pose maybe look up a little bit open up through that throat squeeze those shoulder blades behind and then round down into cat let's add the breath inhale into cow exhaling the cat inhale into cow exhale into calf one more inhale into cow and exhaling the cat and release okay very very good good I'm going to take my right knee and I'm going to cross it over my left leg now if this is uncomfortable for you you can do this one ankle to ankle it's just fine okay so I'm going to take my right hand

and I'm going to place it on the inside of that leg opposite hand is going to come back to the chair lengthen through the spine pull that left shoulder back and then turn and look over that shoulder one more breath here Face Forward take your left hand put it on the outside of the leg opposite hand to the chair lengthen through the spine pull that right shoulder back turn and look and release okay let's uncross our legs and we're going to go to the other side so here we go we're going to cross the

other leg on top or you can be ankle to ankle that's always an option okay left hand on the inside of that thigh opposite hand to the chair lengthen through the spine pull the shoulder back turn and look Face Forward opposite hand comes to the outer thigh opposite other hand to the chair lengthen pull that shoulder back turn and look one more breath and face forward really really good so the next pose is a it's a series that I refer to as swimming so we're going to keep our abdominals tight and this is going to be working into the

back okay so we're going to start with a very small movement and then we'll build into a bigger movement so you're going to listen to your body and do only what works for you all right pull that belly in we're going to just start by pushing see how I'm pushing that arm forward and out and in let's do the other side so I'm leaning forward as I push my arm out swings out and back in let's do it again on the other side all right up we go and we're going to do the other side so we're going to do that one more time

just like this before we add on use your abdominals here you should begin to feel the back working a little bit right as we Lean Forward we're working into that back a little bit and bring those hands down and take a break okay so that's a great version and if that feels good for you you're going to stick with that if you're with me we're going to go a little deeper into that right so we're going to push a little further out and down belly is tight I'm leaning a little bit further forward

and now it's a little bit bigger movement and now we're going to do that again with a little final bigger movement but let's do it one more time like this so this is kind of the medium movement use your abdominals here right protect that back all right and release now if you want to do the full ex extension you're really going to push out belly stays tight but we're really working that back okay here we go push and Center other side push and center switch push come Center and push and Center again push

and push let's do one more on each side working that back last one last side and release okay did that feel did you feel that working through the abdominals to protect that back and you felt that back working and stretching okay good that was the idea okay so now we're going to move into an extended hamstring stretch and we're going to add a pyramid pose okay so I think I don't know a few days ago we did part of this but we're going to add that last little bit onto this series so we're going to bring that right knee in

now remember if you want to hold behind the thigh that's fine okay so you can give that leg a little bit of support here so we're going to flex the foot and we're going to extend now what I want you to do is in lift that leg a little higher oh there's that hamstring you feel it I feel it now you're going to leave your leg long and you're going to ex put that heel on the floor so my leg is straight and long lengthen through the spine hold on to the thighs and let the heart fall forward so we're

adding in that pyramid pose you feel that a little more hamstring here and then tuck the chin and roll it up so the one we did before was a little more quadricep let's bring it up bring that knee in extend so there's the quadricep working but I'm holding on to that leg and I'm going to tug and give that leg a little tug don't lean back right so it's not this it's keeping the spine long there's that hamstring stretch let's put that heel down lengthen and hinge oh I love it boy do you feel that

stretch let's roll it up we're gonna do that one more time bring the knee in Flex the foot extend lift that leg a little higher there's that hamstring oh yeah place the foot on the floor lengthen hinge forward for Pyramid pose oh that feels good and roll it up okay we got to do the other side now are we ready let's bring that knee up and in first so there's a nice little stretch crown of the head long Flex the foot extend lift there's that hamstring place that foot on the floor lengthen

hinge forward for a pyramid pose keep the back flat look out not down and roll it up let's do that again bring that knee in Flex that foot extend the leg now we're going to lift that leg a little higher for that hamstring place a foot on the floor lengthen through the spine hinge forward pyramid pose back is flat and let's do it one more time we got it right bring it in Flex extend lift place the heel on the floor lengthen through the spine let that heart fall forward keeping the back flat for Pyramid pose

and roll it up very very good so we're going to move into goddess pose with shoulder dips we're going to do a little add-on okay so again a heel toe and a heel toe so we've got a nice alignment hips to knees to ankles to toes so everything's in alignment belly stays tight here we're going to hold on to those legs we did this one just a couple of days ago extend nice and long through the spine and we're going to let this shoulder fall down now the difference here what I'm going to do so this shoulder is down I'm going to take this hand and I'm going to press it against that inner thigh so there is the extra stretch so my shoulder dropping is going to get the side waist me pushing into that leg is now getting that inner thigh so it's really kind of adding to this series it's the same series with just a little bit of an add-on here let's come up oh yeah and let's do the other side so let that shoulder fall and then I'm going to press into that leg oh yeah I feel it

one more breath here let's come up can we go straight to the other side let's do it again here we go let that shoulder dip between the legs press against that upper thigh so the inner groin I don't know what all you feel but I'm feeling a lot of stretching going on here and up we go and let's do the other side so by dipping the shoulder I'm feeling the side waist and then as I push it's moving into the inner thigh and the inner groin that's what I personally feel just one more breath here

and let's release that okay go ahead and bring those feet in a little bit so the next stretch again is a pretty intense stretch so it's called the froggy so we're going to sit back in our chair and then we're going to bring our knees out so the seat of the chair is between our legs okay you feel that so let's just hang out here for a couple of breaths and feel that stretch first now whatever feels good for you right if this is just a little too much for you then you're going to go ahead and move

forward and bring those knees in a little it's okay all right extend through the spine nice and long and then just begin to let your heart fall forward so I have my hands on the seat of the chair for support oh yeah all right let's tuck our chin and roll up okay we're going to do that again nice long spine belly tight begin to let your heart fall forward feel the stretch here one more breath tuck the chin and roll it up okay so just bring the legs in a little bit give the uh the inner thighs a little a

little break so as you're resting I want to show you what we're going to do next so we're going to come back the way we were then I'm going to take the heels and I'm going to externally rotate them out it's not a huge movement I don't know if you saw that so I just took my heels from being like at a diagonal here out so that maybe my feet are more 90 degrees toes pointing forward okay so let's all try to do that so go ahead and move back in your chair whatever whatever version of that you're doing

doesn't matter right holding on to that chair now we're going to take our heels and we're going to move them out you'll see how it changes where we're stretching lengthen through the spine pull the belly in let that heart fall forward do you feel the difference right so it's kind of moved the stretch out and around for me anyway oh yeah let's roll it up and we're gonna do that one more time frog inhale extend exhale let the heart fall forward okay so if it feels okay only if you want to I'm going to go

ahead and bring my hands to the floor hi man oh man do y'all feel that stretch just one more breath go ahead and grab your chair okay hold on to that chair roll it up into seated make sure you're not dizzy endless heel toe those feet back in together all right very good so we're gonna do that Warrior Two reverse Warrior side angle pose again but we're going to add a pretty significant stretch for the leg so let's all do the first version 90 degrees just to kind of get it in our head okay then

we're going to go into that pretty deep leg Series so let's take that right knee and open it arms up we've done this one right we've done this one before we're going to look over those front fingertips flip that front Palm to the ceiling reverse your Warrior up and back come back to side to uh Warrior two and then we're going to move to that side angle pose now let's take the hand that's in the air and bring I call it bicep by ear so there is one deepening for this pose that we're going to do

okay pull your belly in and then we're going to begin with this top arm windmill backup to Warrior Two flip that front Palm up and back we're going to move back to that Warrior Two back to side angle remember Hearts lifted we're not letting ourselves sink down bring that bicep by ear oh that feels so good are we ready press into that Warrior Two and release okay so let's bring that knee forward we're going to do that same thing on the other side here we go bring that left knee open 90 degrees between

those legs bring the arms up Warrior Two flip your front Palm up and back we know this one we've done this one a few times right back to that Warrior Two we're going to go to our side angle and then we're going to extend our side angle then I'm going to press back to that Warrior Two flip the Palm up and back back to our Warrior Two side angle pose extended side angle press back to that Warrior Two and release okay excellent so that's a great version and if you want to stick with that version you're going to stick

with that version if you want to be with me what we're going to do is just like we did a minute ago with froggy we're going to bring the seat of the chair between our legs now this leg is pretty much going to stay right where it is okay so it's at a diagonal as everything should be in alignment hips knee ankle and Toes this is the leg that we're going to extend out to the side uh-huh I know I think let's so right here's a couple of things that might happen this happens in my my in-person classes you might be feeling a

little cramped right here so one thing you can do to take some of the pressure off of this upper leg is bend the knee just a smidge okay so that's fine if you want to bend that knee a little bit that's okay but if you're with me I'm going to keep my legs straight I'm up on the side of that foot I'm going to let go of my chair are we ready Warrior Two look over those front fingertips belly tight shoulders are down out of the ears arms are parallel to the mat don't lose the form right

flip the Palm up and back reverse that Warrior side angle pose extended side angle back to Warrior Two flip that Palm up and back back to Warrior Two side angle extended side angle back to Warrior Two reverse your Warrior I know a little flow here back to Warrior Two this is it last one on this side side angle don't let that heart sink extend your side angle press back to Warrior Two hands to the chair bend that extended leg and release I know right that one isn't quite the stretch okay we got to do the other side

so let's come back into that like we were going to do froggy this is a breeze now right you're like we've gone from oh this is a lot to man there's nothing to this piece of it because we've stretched so much in that inner groin okay so we're gonna leave this leg right where it is make sure you're all in alignment now this is the leg that's going to extend I'm up on the side of that leg so I you know just adjust Move Yourself around on that chair until you feel like you've got a position that's going to

work for you okay take a moment here hi remember you can always bend that knee a little bit if that feels better all right bring those arms up look over those left fingertips make sure your shoulders are down those arms are parallel belly is tight are we ready reverse your Warrior Flip that front Palm up and reverse it up to the ceiling I'm looking up if that feels okay on your neck back to Warrior Two side angle pose um let's extend our side angle and press into that Warrior too so let that Palm up and back

back to Warrior Two side angle extend and Warrior two last time through flip that Palm up and back back to Warrior Two side angle reverse I mean extend that side angle back to Warrior Two and release oh bring those legs in right all right so we're going to come to standing and we're going to be on the right side of our chair okay so go ahead and just make sure that you've got that chair handy and we're going to be using it to begin with and then we're not actually I don't think we use it to begin with on this one but you

want to have it here if you need to grab it okay so we're going to come into an extended standing mountain pose so belly is tight right shoulders are down interlace your fingers Point your fingers to the ceiling now we're going to lean our Mountain towards our chair so keep that this foot down all right so feel that stretch and then we're going to come up and then we're going to lean the other way and then we're going to come up and let's bring those hands down so just checking in how does that feel so what

we're going to do is as we lean towards our chair we're going to lift this leg up all right so we're going to do a little bit of balance but we're only going to do it on that one side and then we'll go to the other side of the chair because I want you leaning in towards the chair because you can grab it if you need to all right ready extended Mountain we got this shoulders down interlace I mean bring your palms together interlace fingers pointer finger to the ceiling okay so let's start just leaning to the mountain keep

your feet on the floor for right now then we're going to come up and we're going to lean the other way okay are we ready we're going to come up now lean towards your your chair let's extend that leg Out start with your toes down then see if you can lift that foot up I know right quite the balance challenge in three two one bring the leg down and bring the hands down let's do the other side so a balanced challenge where we're moving and leaning is a very challenging all right so here we go we've got both

feet on the floor we're going to come into that extended Mountain Palms together interlace fingers pointer finger to the ceiling we're going to lean towards our chair and up we go and we're going to lean the other way and up we go and let's lean towards our chair let's take that foot that left foot come up to the toes first then we're going to lift that leg up leaning Mountain with one leg I know right one more breath up we go and release excellent work all right turn and face your chair so the leg next to the back of the chair

I want you to set that foot under the chair so that when you bend your knee your knee or your shin touches the chair take your back leg and we're going to bring it back at that 45 degree angle so bend that front knee bring your hips around a little bit to face me and come into that Warrior Two shoulders are down belly is tight make sure your ribs are in the center of the body so this is our front hand we're going to flip that Palm to the ceiling we're going to reverse our Warrior up and back come back to your Warrior Two now the

right hand is going to come down into the chair opposite heart arm extends out look up a little bit if that feels okay so make sure your shoulder shoulder and wrist are in alignment now if you want to extend you can extend don't worry if you don't want to do that part don't worry about it all right belly tight are we ready come into Warrior Two let's do that again flip that Palm up and back back to Warrior Two hand to the chair side angle pose extend that side angle press it up into that Warrior too

squeeze the muscles against the bones in the arms right activate that upper body and release okay good let's come to the other side okay so again placing that foot under the chair right bending that knee so that that knee touches the chair take a step back with that back foot that back heel is down bend the front knee and rotate those hips around to face me arms are out so there we are in our beautiful Warrior Two make sure your ribs are in the center of the body shoulders are down look over those front fingertips flip

that front Palm up and back reverse that Warrior come back to that Warrior Two hand comes to the chair side angle pose extend that arm over by set by ear press up into your Warrior Two flip that Palm up and back back to Warrior Two hand in the chair side angle pose arm up and over last time through it we got this Warrior Two reverse it side angle pose extended side angle press up activate the upper body squeeze the muscles against the bones in those arms and release excellent very very good okay so this is going to be a heart opener

with eagle arms so you're going to be buyer's chair but make sure that you're not going to hit the chair when you move your hands all right so maybe just a little further forward let's clasp our hands behind our back press the knuckles down and Away open up through that chest one more breath here bring the arms wide press those arms back there open up through that heart squeeze those shoulder blades behind now we're going to cross we're going to take that right arm on top so you've got one elbow

stacked on top of the other we're going to bounce three times now we're going to give ourselves a hug we're going to lift our elbows up on an inhale and we're going to bring them forward and down on an exhale inhale come up open those arms squeeze your shoulder blades back behind you and Let's cross the other arm on top bounce bounce bounce grab your shoulders give yourself a hug inhale lift exhale down elbows are coming down towards the floor lift those elbows up let's open we're going to switch sides one more

time bounce bounce bounce now if you want your arms are going to go up follow your elbows with your gaze and then I want you to open your arms up into star pose up until those tippy toes come back down hug yourself the other way elbows up inhale elbows down exhale elbows up on an inhale open up into star pose your arms are up at a v come up onto those tippy toes you're looking up shoulders are down belly is tight one more breath and down we go how did you do on that one right I know there's kind of a lot of moving parts for that

whole series I hope that you were able to follow I hope I cued it well for you all right so we're going to take our right knee we came to seated I don't even think I said that I just sat down but I didn't tell you what I was doing so we've returned to our seated position and we're going to move into half lord of the fishes so we're going to take our right knee and we're going to open it that left arm is going to open nice and wide and we're going to bring it all the way across our body we're going to grab

the chair lift through the crown of the head turn and look over the back of your chair hold and breathe let's open up and do that again bring that arm all the way across the body grab the chair lift the crown of the head towards the ceiling turn and look over the back of your chair and release let's go ahead and face forward and we're going to do the other side so we're going to open ride our opens up and then it comes across the body we grab the chair lift turn and look over the back of that

chair let's release that I'll open that arm again bring it all the way across your body grab the chair lift and twist and face forward okay so we're going to move into pigeon pose you can cross ankle to ankle or you can cross ankle to knee hang out here for just a moment Rod feeling the stretch right in here lifting nice and long through the spine if you wish let that heart fall forward oh yeah there's a good stretch hip and glute tuck the chin and roll it up let's move that knee up and down just a little

bit and we're going to do that again extending long through the spine belly tight let that heart fall forward pigeon pose uh and let's switch sides okay so you've got that ankle to ankle version if that one that one works better for you or ankle to knee just hang out here for a couple of breaths feeling the stretch to begin with then we're going to lengthen through the spine and we're going to let our heart fall forward keep that back flat look out not down tuck the chin and roll it up and then

let's move that knee up and down just a little bit and we're gonna do that one more time nice long spine inhale exhale as you come forward keeping the back flat looking out not down there's that stretch for the hip and glute I one more breath and uh really good place that foot on the floor and we're gonna get ready for shavasana pose so our relaxing pose at the end of our practice so if you want to sit back and lean back on the chair go for it hands resting lightly on the thighs let's flip

the Palms up close your eyes take a deep breath in and a full breath out embrace the difficulty make the problem any less problematic by hiding from it embrace the difficulty and you begin to give yourself a measure of control over it exercise your courage and improve your effectiveness at the same time admit the shortcomings limitations mistakes and disappointments then do something about them you're not going to fool anybody by pretending there's not a problem what you can do is impress everyone

including yourself by meeting the problem head on look at the situation with Clarity and with the highest expectations throw in a little humor and good cheer ask yourself what would turn a negative into a positive from what areas within this challenge with what specific actions can you extract opportunity and value look honestly and bravely at the pro what you'll see is a chance to add new richness to life feel your courage take hold as you embrace the difficulty and transform it into something good take a deep breath in

and a full breath out drop your right ear towards your right shoulder reach up with the right hand give the head a gentle hug pressing that opposite hand down towards the floor release it drop your chin towards your chest reaching up with the hands giving the head a gentle tug release it drop your left ear towards your left shoulder reach up with the left hand give the head a gentle tug pressing that opposite arm down towards the floor release it look up just slightly open your mouth if you want to stretch your jaw bring your hands to your heart

DAY 25

I'm glad you joined me today so today today is day 25 wow of our 28 day chair yoga journey together so we're gonna start seated with the cow face pose we'll go to standing and then we'll come back to seated so in our for our cow face foes and a couple of other poses we're going to use a strap today so if you don't have a strap you can substitute a necktie or a scarf you can do it without it it's fine I'll show you how to do that but if you have it it's kind of Handy to use it for a few of the poses that we're going to be doing today okay so remember I'd love for you to click the Subscribe button it is free and leave me a comment all right so we're going to get started now we're going to move forward in our chair and make sure that we're not leaning back so think about crown of the head lifts up shoulders are down out of the ears let's take a moment to ground our feet to the Earth pulling that belly button in towards the

spine let's ground our sits and Bones to the chair lift your heart lower your shoulders place your hands lightly on your thighs flip the Palms up to the ceiling close your eyes connect to your heart center notice your natural breath just feeling your inhalation and exhalation move that breath down into the diaphragm as you inhale the belly extends we're filling the lungs from the bottom up and as we exhale we're actively pulling the belly button in towards the spine and pushing the air up and out of the

lungs do that a couple of times and breathe normally bring your hands to your heart set your intentions for today's practice focusing in on what you want to accomplish one more breath here bring your hands back down to your thighs and open your eyes let's look to the right and look Center look to the left and Center we're going to do that again so as you look to the right see if you can take your gaze a little bit further just feeling the natural stretch here so we're not trying to overdo it right so

it's a gentle thing here go ahead and look Center and let's look at the other side just trying to engage a little deeper into that stretch taking your gaze a little further over the shoulder and very very good so we're going to drop our hands towards the floor and we're going to shrug our shoulders up into our ears and then we're going to drop them down and we're going to do that again shrug drop one more shrug and drop wow very good so drop your right ear towards your right shoulder reach up at the right hand and you're

just going to lay that hand lightly on the head just feel a little extra stretch there you're not pulling or tugging just letting the weight of the hand give you a little extra stretch High one more breath take the hand off lift the head up and let's go to the other side so we're going to drop that ear to shoulder first so feel that stretch to begin with then we're going to reach up with the hand and you're just going to lay it lightly on that head don't pull or tug ah one more breath take your hand off of

the head and lift that head up excellent excellent work so we're going to move into some pelvic tilts here to warm up that spine so we're going to take our hip tips and rot them towards our shoulders so feel that rotation right that that tilting forward the shoulders are kind of coming forward the hips are back now we're going to take those hip tips and rock them towards our shoulders so it's kind of the opposite so we're lifting up through our chest and that back is making a little bit of

an arch and let's do that again hands can be just on the thighs for a little support if you like that and then up we go and we're going to do that one more time and lift it up and release all right excellent work so we're going to move into our Mountain pose so we're going to take those hands down spread those fingers wide shoulders are out of the ears belly is tight goal post arms squeeze behind extend your hands to the ceiling shoulders or down belly is tight extended Mountain bring the hands down so we're going to

do that one more time bring those hands down go post arms squeeze your shoulder blades back behind you and now let's extend that mountain all right bring the hands down so now we're going to do that extended Mountain in series but we're going to add a little strap so go ahead and grab that strap or your necktie or your scarf and if you're doing it without it just mimic having the strap in your hand it's fine so what I want you to do is double up that strap Okay so we've we've doubled

it up just to make it a little bit shorter and then I want you to grab the straps in each hand and I don't know you know 18 inches between the hands something like that okay we're going to bring those hands up to the ceiling all right so shoulders stay down belly stays tight so here we are in our extended Mountain just like we did a minute ago but we've got this strap now and you'll see we'll be adding some things in using that strap okay so the first thing we're going to do is just a normal leaning Mountain

now we're leaning here so make sure you're keeping that opposite hip down right so keeping the hips down and then come up and then we're going to lean our Mountain the other way and then we're going to come up and we're going to do that again let's lean our Mountain and come up and we're going to lean our Mountain the other way oh boy come up go ahead and bring those hands down and take just a little break how's that feeling let's roll those shoulders a little bit okay all right really good so now we're going

to do that again and with one uh add-on and you don't have to add on right so let's come back up into our extended Mountain okay we're going to lean our Mountain to the right now what I want you to do is take your left hand and I want you to bring it over so that the strap is parallel to the mat so belly is tight or you feel your side waist muscles working pretty hard here right belly tight let's take that arm back up to the ceiling and we're going to come up and then we're going to lean the other way

now the other arm the right arm is going to come down that strap is parallel to the mat belly is tight bring that arm back up come back up to the hands to the ceiling bring the arms down take a break we're going to do that one more time oh my nose is itching sorry okay so ready here we go extending we're going to lean to the left this time first then we're going to take that right arm and we're going to bring it down so that the strap is parallel to the mat belly is tight working your side waist muscles

all right let's take that twist out come up we're going to go to the other side so that we lean the mountain first then we're going to twist and then we're going to bring that arm back up to remove the twist bring the arms up and release okay did that feel all right good so we're gonna come into a seated cow face pose and we're going to take our strap and we're going to put it in our right hand okay so you've got your strap it's just going to kind of hang here in that hand and I

want you to bring the Palm to Face Forward now what you're going to do is you're going to bend your elbow okay so you see kind of see what I'm doing there I'm still holding my my strap I'm going to bend my elbow and I'm going to bring it so the upper my palm is in the upper part of my back and my strap is hanging down okay so just we're bending That Elbow and then bringing that back that strap back behind okay now your other arm your palm is going to face back now when you bend that elbow see that uh

the arm's coming down now you're going to bring that hand back behind you and you're going to grab that strap back behind you okay so I've got the top of the strap in one hand I've got the bottom of the strap in the other hand lift up through the heart squeeze so I want your elbows back you're kind of pulling on that strap for a little extra stretch lift through the heart we're holding and we're breathing one more breath all right let's release that oh have that feet on I know right

what the stretch okay we're gonna do the other side okay so my arm I mean my hand is facing forward and I've just got the strap in my hand no it's facing back isn't it I'm sorry facing back now it's facing forward I was right it's facing forward all right so we're going to bend that elbow we're going to bring that hand and we're going to place it into the top of the back and that strap is just hanging behind me now the other hand is going to be facing back so when you bend that elbow right

you're hinging here now bring that hand to the small of the back and grab the strap so elbows are back see how I'm pressing my elbows back lifting up through the heart now pull gently on that strap and to give yourself a little extra stretch I will tell you if you have shoulder issues this might be a little too much so just listen to your body do what feels good for you right we have one more breath and release huh let's roll those shoulders it's quite a stretch okay really really good all right so

we're going to move into seated hand to toe pose and we're going to be using our strap if you don't have your strap you're just going to be using your hands so what will happen is we're going to lift that foot and extend the leg and you'll just be using your hand to toe so hand to toe pose right that kind of makes sense what I like about having the strap or the necktie or the scarf is it just extend your hands a little bit and I think for me personally it's really hard to be in this pose with good form it's

just a little too much for me so what I'm going to do is I'm going to put my strap on the floor and then I'm going to set the ball of my right foot into that strap I'm going to hold one side of the strap in each hand and then I'm going to bring my foot out let's start with knee bent a little bit okay get the nice long spine crown of the head to the ceiling pull your belly in super tight and let's extend that leg so maybe do a little bicep curl and lengthen that hamstring a little bit

so how does that feel oh yeah one more breath let's bend that knee and put that foot down and we're going to go to the other side so just a little hamstring stretch to start with so put the ball of the foot into the strap and then bend that knee up so here's the thing I didn't say on the other side you want to make sure the strap is on the ball of the foot and not the arch okay I've got the one strap in each hand in that ball of the foot so the art let's go ahead and extend that leg while I

talk and then just pull up just a little bit don't lean back belly tight so we've got a lot of really small bones in the arches of the feet and we don't really want the strap to be pulling on that part of the body we want it to be on this ball of the foot it can handle it okay we're going to bend that knee and put that foot there okay so we kind of got the feeling of it now so the we're going to be adding a couple of things on and remember do what feels good for you I'll cue it and if you

don't want to do that part leave it out all right so let's go back to that right foot so we're going to put the ball of the right foot in bend the knee and extend the leg let's give it just a little bicep curl I know right so I'm saying bicep curl it's just because that's kind of what what's happening with my arms from my leg to extend up crown of the head to the ceiling now what I want you to do is grab the straps in your left hand now your right hand can come to the chair don't lean back don't round keep the

heart lifted crown of the head to the ceiling we're going to bring that leg across the midline of the body so this is what you should be feeling stretching right here okay so now grab the stress in that other hand opposite hand to the chair and open oh my goodness there's that groin stretch right you feel it and we're going to come Center grab the strap come across the body come center now here's the little add-on hold that chair so you're going to bend this right knee now I'm letting this strap go a little

bit in my hand I'm sliding it down and I'm going to bring that knee down by the chair so this is a seated dancer pose okay pretty good stretch for this side one more breath and let's release that okay so let's go to the other side and then the final add-on is the seated dancer but we're going to let go of the chair but we got to do a couple of things before we do that okay so let's go ahead and place the left ball of the foot in the chair I've got one strap in each hand and I'm

going to lift up I'm going to choke up just a little bit here okay now I'm going to extend that leg along give it a little tug grab the straps in the right hand left hand to chair bring that leg across the body hand to toe pose all right now bring that leg Center grab the other hand we're going to open do you notice how I've let go of the chair and I've extended this arm out there's an add-on if you want to do that it's a little balance work too belly tight okay so now bring that foot forward

slide so I'm going to slide that strap the hand up the straps I'm going to bend this knee bring the straps up and over the shoulder for a seated dancer pose one more breath okay so let's release that now what I want to do is I want to just do the dancer part of that because I want to move a little bit to the side so we can drop that knee down better so let's move a little bit to the right side of our chair okay so I call this one cheek on and One Cheek off so I'm going to put my right foot into

the strap then I'm going to pull that strap up over my shoulder and I'm going to hold that chair for right now so this see how much further that knee can fall down now because I've moved over and there's space now for that knee to drop you should be feeling the quadricep stretching all right if it feels good for you you're gonna pull that belly in super tight and you're going to let go of that chair oh there's your beautiful seated dancer pose we have one more breath bring your hand back down to

the chair and really ha okay we gotta do the other side now ready let's come to the other side my left foot is right in the hook of that strap we're going to pull that strap up over our shoulder that knee is falling down towards the floor belly is tight okay we ready we're gonna let go of the chair and we're gonna extend there's your dancer pose belly tight for three two and one let's hang on to that chair and we're going to release all right very good let's go ahead and just set

our strap down under our chair out of our way and we're going to move into a series here we're going to work a little bit into the shoulders and the legs so I'm moving a little bit forward in my chair and then what I'm going to do is I'm going to bring my arms parallel I'm going to do a half shoulder press up to the ceiling and then down and let's do the other side it's just a half shoulder press up and down now we're going to add a heel lift so the same side the heel of the same side is lifting up and down so

as I'm doing my half shoulder press my heel is coming up and bringing it down let's do that again one more on each side you know we're adding on and uh and down so now see if it feels okay for a full shoulder press now if that's too much on your shoulders let's go to the other side you're going to stick with that half shoulder press okay it's okay just listen to your body let's do that again how's that feeling and down one more on the other side okay now instead of a heel lift we're going to lift our knee same knee of the leg of the arm that's extending so we're doing the same side as what I'm trying to say I didn't say that very well did I and down let's do that again full extension knee is lifting and down your alternative is half shoulder press with the heel remember you don't have to add on let's do one more on each side last one last side and release excellent work okay grab your strap come to standing on the right side of your chair all right so if you don't have your strap what you're going to do is again you'll be doing hand to toe pose here it's it's a pretty challenging series I encourage you to go in and hold on to the chair and maybe you'll need to bend the knee a little bit I would rather you keep your heart lifted and bend the knee a little bit then get the legs straight and be hunched over okay does that make sense but if you're with me we're going to use our handy dandy strap or our necktie or our scarf and then I'm going to put so I've got one side of the strap in

each hand and then I'm going to place the kind of that bottom this of the strap onto the floor and let's start with our right foot okay so it's not the leg next to the chair that's the leg that's going to give us the support okay so the other leg is the one that I'm stepping into the strap now I'm going to go ahead and I'm going to choke up a little bit I'm going to move my hand down the strap let's bend the knee to begin with hold on to that chair extend that leg excellent work okay notice how high my

heart is lifted my crown of the head is to the ceiling I'm not leaning forward I'm not hunched over let's bring that leg across the body place that foot into the seat of the chair for just a moment oh there's a stretch you feel that okay lift the leg we're going to come and we're going to open it up oh yeah hold that chair this isn't balanced don't worry about the balance yet let's come forward let's put that foot back into the seat of the chair now go ahead and open up that so I'm

moving my hand up on the strap a little bit because we're going to move into a dancer pose and you're going to want to have more length of that strap okay so come forward now bend your knee break the knee down towards the opposite knee and the strap comes up and over your back so the key to this particular series is trying to get that knee down so often what I'll see is kind of this right so the idea is to try to get the bent knee down as close to the standing knee as you can pull that belly in super tight

can you let go of the chair and bring that hand up into a dancer pose one more breath bring your hand back down to the chair and release excellent work okay let's go to the other side okay so remember we've got one strap in each hand knot the foot next to the chair the other one we're going to step the ball of the foot into the into the bottom of that strap we're going to choke up a little bit of your left hand choke it up hold that chair with that right lift that foot up nice long spine belly tight

we're going to bring that foot across the body place the foot into the seat of the chair lift and open up that hand to toe pose oh my goodness let's do that again bring it across the body place the heel into the seat of the chair okay let's go ahead and slide our hand up that strap just a little bit we're going to bring that knee across now we're going to bend the knee bring the strap up and over that shoulder and again trying to let that knee fall down towards the opposite knee just hang out here let that happen right so just

breathe into the stretch let that quadricep on that of this side right so this is the quadricep that you're going to be stretching let that feel there you go all right so the little bit of balance here we're going to pull that belly in super tight ready let go of the chair extend the arm out Palm faces up there's your dancer pose one more breath go ahead and grab the chair and release excellent very good you guys okay so I'm gonna keep my uh strap doubled and I'm going to Tang my feet a good

solid hip distance apart maybe a little further now I'm going to grab my one strap and all right in each hand about I don't know what 18 inches apart and I'm going to bring my hands up to the ceiling so you want your arms to be at a v right so whatever feels good for you it's okay belly's going to be tight so we're going to lean in towards our chair and then it's come up and then we're going to lean the other way and we're going to come up now we're going to lean towards our chair and

we're going to let our outside arm come forward so keep the elbows straight the strap is parallel to the mat bring that elbow arm back up hands overhead and let's go the other way so we're going to lean first then we're going to let this outside arm dip down bring that arm back up and up we go one more time on each side lean little twist here bring that arm up and up we go we're going to lean the other way arm comes down I don't know about you but boy I feel this up we go belly tight uh up we go and everything's

again doesn't look like we're doing much but boy I feel that one okay let's just put our strap under our chair and kind of get it out of our way so we're going to move into a plank pose now while you're playing I'm going to give you lots of options here so everybody can be successful in a plank pose I know right everybody but what I do want to encourage you is to make sure your chair is on a carpet or a sticky mat like a yoga mat something that's not going to slide we are definitely going

to consciously think about pressing down and not out but I'd rather you have that chair stable to make sure it's not going to slide out from under you all right so we're going to turn and we're going to face our chair and we're going to take the leg next to the back of the chair and we're going to place that foot under the chair so that when we Bend our knee we can feel that uh leg touching the chair now you're going to bring your your other foot out back behind you now I don't care if you want to turn that heel

in and and have that at an angle it's fine if you want to have it I'll tend to all toes pointing forward that's fine too I'm going to let you choose the version because this isn't about stretching that back leg right this is not what this is about so that belly so abdominals are going to be working really really hard here as well as the upper body okay all right so we're going to pull that belly in and we're going to hinge forward and place your hands in the chair all right now you're going to bend your

elbows and you're going to place those forearms in the seat of the chair all right so what we've done here let's bend that front knee a little bit more is we're in a plank position but we've got some support because that front leg is there giving us that support right you feeling that so I'm going to look down at my chair I'm going to take a deep breath in and on an exhale I'm going to go ahead and come up now what we're going to do is as we come down we're going to be on those forearms

and if you want you're going to take this front foot back into a plank if you want to leave the front foot on the floor that's fine it's just a supported plank all right are we ready let's do it bend that front knee hinge forward place the hands in the chair first now we're just going to bend those elbows so our forearms are in the chair okay I'm looking down I'm gonna pull my belly in super tight I'm pressing down not out inhale exhale bring that foot back forearm plank okay so I'm looking down

my the pressure is on my forearms I don't want the pressure on the elbows so bring that weight forward just a little bit pressing down into those forearms your belly is pulling in make sure those hips are lower I just felt that my hips were a little high so I'm going to lower my hips a little bit so you want the shoulders the hips the ankles all in alignment are you feeling it I know I'm feeling it too pull that belly in okay for three two one now to come out of it bring that foot back forward other foot forward

roll it up and come into standing okay how's that feel can we do the other side so let's come to the other side of our chair I'm going to move my strap just a little bit out of my way so the foot next to the chair is the one that's going to come forward make sure you can bend that knee and you can touch the chair okay now the other leg is going to step back remember you can have that heel down at an angle or it can be down with the toe straight it doesn't matter either is fine but I want you to bend that front knee

make sure you can touch the chair with the knee so you're close enough to the chair all right pull your belly in hinge forward place the hands in the seat of the chair bend your elbows go ahead and put those forearms in the seat of the chair okay so I'm looking down I'm feeling this is my my belly is tight this is our supported plank pose okay so we're going to go straight in to the full plank we kind of know what we're doing now all right are we ready we're going to inhale to prepare and as we exhale we're going to bring

that front foot back bring that weight forward make sure the weight is on the forearms right knob the elbows so I'm kind of pulling back in my my heels so that's going to help you also think about getting the hips down a little bit so my belly is super tight here in my plank pose I'm looking down at the at the mat if that feels okay or in the seat of the chair is what I should say so belly is super tight here I'm not grasping that that chair with my hands right they're loose my fingers are loose here the

weight is in this in the forearms and I've just got a couple more breaths I know my belly's shaking too one more breath bring your legs foot forward first other leg comes forward and roll it up I didn't say that very clearly oh my goodness let's come to seated so how are you feeling on that one to get your heart rate up a little bit that was challenging I know that it is so let's do a little stretching I should feel good let's take that right knee and open it wide we're going to let that

left knee fall down towards the floor push the foot back lift the heart okay just taking a couple of breaths here feeling a nice stretch in our Crescent lunge let's release the knee and then we're going to press that kneecap up towards the ceiling we're really warm we can give that a little extra stretch all right let's face forward now let's grab our strap again if you've got it we're going to put it's our left leg so the same leg we were just working in that Crescent lunge let's put the strap

around the ball of the foot and I've got one strap in each hand lengthen nice and long through the spine I'm going to pull gently a little flexion of that foot and then let that heart fall forward into pyramid pose so it's a little assisted pyramid pose might give you a little additional stretch keep the back flat look out not down tuck the chin and roll it up and let's do that one more time nice long spine exhale as we come down pulling gently on that leg and release just set the strap in your

lap we'll come back to it for the other side let's come into our pigeon pose ankle to ankle is fine ankle to knee if you feels okay lengthen nice and long through the spine and let that heart fall forward there's that hit stretch for those that hip glute area right feels so good tuck the chin and roll it up let's move that knee a little up and down we're gonna do that again nice long spine heart Falls forward and up we go okay let's do the other side so we're going to take this left

knee and open it right knee falls down towards the floor push that foot back if that feels okay back of the kneecap to the ceiling relax into this glute nice long spine release it let the knee fall down towards the mat and then we'll do that again and phase four let's use our strap again we're going to strap put the strap around the ball of that foot one hand in each strap lengthen nice and long through the spine pull so their little calf stretch to begin with then let that heart fall forward so I'm just pulling gently on

that foot to give me a little extra stretch and Tuck the chin and roll it out let's do that one more time nice long spine inhale exhale forward and release go ahead and unhook the strap set it down come into your pigeon pose so you can do the ankle to ankle version if you like that one you can do the ankle to knee version if you prefer that one nice long spine and heart Falls forward tuck that chin and roll it up and we're going to do that one more time extending long heart Falls forward oh that feels so good

and roll it I I forgot to move that needless to move the knee just a little nice little movement for that hip joint okay we're gonna move into shavasana Palms Lean Back hands resting lightly on the thighs flip the Palms up to the ceiling take a deep breath in and as you exhale go ahead and close the eyes steps available to you you have the ability you have the opportunity you have resources transform them into value your needs will not be met by merely focusing on those needs to satisfy your needs and desires you must do what you can do with whatever you have you can't do everything yet you can do something conditions are not perfect yet they do present you with certain opportunities within the limitations within the restraints within the challenges those very real opportunities exist seek to find them to focus on them and to act on them wishing for things to be easier will only make things harder so spend your energy on productive action rather than on empty wishes or toxic resentments there is a path from here to where you

need to be take the steps available to you and put yourself solidly on that path take a deep breath in and a full breath out drop the right ear towards the right shoulder reach up with the right hand give the head a gentle tug pressing that left hand down towards the floor release it drop your chin towards your chest reach up with the hands give the head a gentle tug release it drop your left ear towards your left shoulder reach up with the left hand give the head a gentle time pressing that right hand down towards the floor release it look out just slightly open your mouth if you want to stretch your jaw bring your hands to your heart

DAY 26

we're going to move forward in our chair nice long spine right we're not leaning back crown of the head to the ceiling hands are resting lightly on the thighs flip those Palms up let's take a moment to ground our feet to the floor and our sits bones to the chair close our eyes draw your attention inward toward your heart center noticing your breath your inhalation and exhalation we're going to move that breath down into the diaphragm as we inhale the belly extends feeling those lungs up from the bottom up and as we exhale actively pull the belly button in towards the spine pushing the air up and out of the lungs

do that a couple more times and breathe normally bring your hands to your heart set your intentions for today's practice one more breath here bring your hands back down to your thighs and open your eyes roll those shoulders forward up back and down let's do that again forward up back and down and reverse it back up forward down one more back up forward and down very very good okay so we're going to extend our Mountain fingertips towards the ceiling shoulders are down belly is tight so with our right hand we're going to grab our left

wrist we're going to lengthen it up towards the ceiling and then we're going to lean oh yeah that should feel good and then we're gonna come up and we're going to grab the other wrist and we extend it up towards the ceiling first and then lean and up we go let's release that and we're going to do that just one more time okay extend that mountain now the left hand grabs the right wrist lengthen and hinge and then lean come up grab that other wrist lengthen and lean up we go bring the hands down and

release let's do another shoulder roll all right and release it and do it the other way and release okay really good so we're going to grab the back of our chair lift that heart up squeeze the shoulder blades behind you and come into that cowl pose and then we're going to take our hands round them place the hands on the thighs round the back tuck the chin let the head fall and come into your calf pose looking at your belly button not hold don't hold the head up here okay let's inhale and come into cow

and exhale and come into cat inhale into cow exhale into cat one more time inhale into cow and exhaling the calf and release all right so we're going to start with our right leg and we're going to ham our hand under that thigh and we're going to lift that knee up Flex the foot extend the leg place the heel on the floor lengthen through the spine and let the heart fall forward nice tuck the chin and roll it up hand under the thigh same leg bend the knee bring that thigh in nice long spine belly tight Flex the foot extend the leg

place the foot on the floor lengthen and hinge okay we're going to do a little add-on here so we're going to reach underneath bend that knee up now we're going to let go of the leg extend place the heel on the floor lengthen and hinge let's do that again roll it up bend the knee don't hold if you can if that works okay if you need to hold that spine belly tight Flex the foot extend now we're going to hold for three and two and one bend that knee and put that foot on the floor whoa yeah feel the quads

working a little right belly stays tight okay we're gonna go the other side so we're gonna bring that knee up let's hold first okay nice long spine Flex the foot extend place the heel on the floor lengthen through the spine let the heart fall forward tuck the chin roll it up bend the knee grab behind the thigh bring that foot up Flex the foot extend place the heel on the floor lengthen hinge forward tuck the chin and roll it up bend that knee Flex the foot extend the leg heel to the floor lengthen and lean forward

tuck the chin and roll it up okay here we go with the add-on let's lift that leg up don't hold on Flex extend place the heel on the floor lengthen hinge forward last time we've got this ready roll it up here we go bend the knee lift up Flex extend now hold for three and two and one bend the knee and put the foot on the floor excellent excellent work okay so I'm going to bring my arms up my forearms are parallel to one another and then I'm going to bring one arm out and then I'll bring it in

and let's bring the other arm out and Center let's do that again out and Center out and Center okay belly tied we're going to add the legs okay here we go outer inner thigh abdominals engaged and centered and let's do the other side you got it and center arm opens as the leg opens and Center and open let's do one more on each side we've got it and Center last one last Side open and Center all right very very good so hands are going to rest on those thighs and we're going to do some body circles

so let's start to the right come Center to the left and back and to the right Center left now stop and let's reverse it okay so we're going to the left first Center right back let's do one more like that then we're going to have we have one little add-on here all right very good go ahead and come back up to seated so that's a great version having your hands on your thighs is great because it gives you some support now if you're with me we're going to not have our hands on the thighs we're going to like have our

hands here like we're going to stir a big old pot okay we're gonna go forward big circles out and back outside forward there's your back you feel it keep those abdominals engaged working all the muscles here and let's reverse it so our side waist muscles are working our back is working our abdominals are working it's really good for all the muscles in the center of the Body for the core and release all right excellent work now a few days ago we did a sun salutation with the bead which adds that

chair pose what we're going to add on today is some twisting okay so if it doesn't work for your back you're just going to stay in chair pose you don't have to do the twists all right so we're going to start with just a normal Sun salutation just to get to get the feeling of it we'll add in that chair pose and then we'll add those twists all right so hands to Heart we're going to take a big circle up hands over head Mountain pose bring your hands to Heart we're going to inhale as

we come up and then we're going to forward salute with our plane arms and extend those arms back behind you nice long spine hands on those thighs Palms face up there's your supported forward fold tuck the chin roll it up bring your hands to your heart let's do that again before we add on big old Circle up we got a mountain pose bring your hands to Heart back to Mountain pose we go dive forward forward salute airplane arms supported forward fold now from here we're going to take our hands to our

heart we're going to act like we're going to get out of the chair but we're not belly tight activate those quadriceps and the abdominals and release okay are we ready now this time we're going to actually lift our hips up out of the chair so make sure your feet are in a position so when you press down you can lift your hips up hands to Heart let's do it big circle up we go Mountain pose bring your hands to Heart we're going to come back to Mountain pose and we're going to dive forward forward salute airplane arm

stretch now bring your hands to your heart inhale to prepare exhale come into your chair pose all right now here we are in chair pose belly is tight hips are back knees are bent knees are behind the toes I want you to be able to wiggle those toes right heart is lifted inhale to prepare we're going to twist to the right now everybody look down at that knee this knee needs to not come forward all right so if this knee is forward you're twisting at the hips I want the hips to stay forward the knees to stay forward

the action to happen right at the rib cage we're going to come Center and then we're going to twist the other way we're holding and we're breathing we're going to come back Center we're going to have a seat and we're going to return to our starting position big circle up we go Mountain pose bring your hands to heart back up to Mountain pose we go forward salute our plane arms let's stretch let's do that supported forward fold bring your hands to your heart in how to prepare exhale up we go

okay are we ready inhale exhale we're going to twist the other way first this time making sure those knees are forward just take a peek at them right make sure this knee is not coming forward let's come Center and then we're going to twist the other way we're going to come Center we're going to have a seat and we're going to get ready now we're going to have one final add-on all right big circle up we go Mountain pose bring your hands to Heart back to Mountain pose we go forward salute airplane arms stretch

hands to Heart inhale to prepare exhale come up into chair pose okay so now we're going to twist to the right the add-on here is we're going to open our wingspan so this hand is on the outside of this leg as we extend and that gives us an opportunity to twist a little deeper only if that works for you okay bring your hands back to Heart come back Center this is it we're going to twist the other way we're going to open that wingspan if you want to one more breath here bring your hands back to Heart Take the twist out have a

seat and take a break very very good okay so now we're going to move into boat pose so I'm moving forward in my chair all right I'm going to hold my chair and then I'm going to lift my right knee up off the floor and then down and left up and down left up and down right up and down right up and down left up and down left up and down right up and down and take just a little break so I'm playing with your brain a little bit too aren't I so we have a little bit of a cueing with the brain

working so you know if it doesn't work for you just it's fine just lift them over okay so now I'm gonna do that but I'm not going to hold on all right so I'm going to bring my Palms out my Palms are facing up my arms are added to the diagonal lifting up and here we go up and down other side up and down left up and down right up and down right up and down left up and down left up and down right up and down and take a break so how did that feel okay all right so we're going to hold that

chair lifting up nice and Tall belly tight we're going to lift one knee then we're going to lift the other knee so here's the thing I'm going to turn to the side you stay facing me what I want you to think about is pelvic tilt okay so hip tips to shoulder a little pelvic tilt lift and lift so I'm balancing up on that tailbone shoulders are down all right so you kind of see what I'm doing there a little balance now what we're going to do is we're going to drop our toes so instead of lifting we're

here balanced you can hold that chair if you want to or you can let go shoulders are down let's bring our foot down and up and down and up down and up and down and up again down and up down and up down and up other side down and up and take a break oh how's that feel let's do a little cat and cow here lifting up through the spine and rounding that back okay so a little cat Cow here nice long spine everybody feeling okay and round it down so remember we're building and we're adding right so

you've got lots of versions that you can do you can do any of them you don't have to keep building and adding it's okay all right if you're with me here we go we're going to hold on first let's get one leg up in the other let's find our balance so make sure you're lifting up I don't want I mean there's a little bit of a of a of a rounding that happens right so I want you to feel like you're rounding and not you know I don't know how to describe it but what I'll see in

my classes is people right here right other gents in their turn if you'll just pull that belly in and round a little bit that's going to give you more balance okay hold the chair if you want let go if you don't now instead of down and up we're going to go up so this leg we're going to take Lick It Up and down other side up and down up and down up and down up and down up and down last time both sides up and down put your feet on the floor pray pray I know I feel it too okay so the very last thing we're going

to do is a roll in of our boat so we'll start hands at heart I want you to extend your right leg out and I want you to twist to the left maybe that left elbow comes to the floor maybe or to the chair maybe it doesn't and up we go let's do the other side extend twist and up switch sides so the leg is extending I'm twisting and Center last time like this and up we go okay so that's an excellent version if you want to stick with that version please do so the very last thing if you're with me I'm going to come up into that balanced position I'm going to bring my hands to my heart now I'm going to extend the leg and twist but I'm balanced and then up extend the other side and twist and up extend and twist and up extended twist and up can we do one more on each side I know I'm feeling it two and up last one last side and up and release let's do a cat Cow here nice and long maybe bring those arms to the back wall thumbs to the back wall and round we're gonna do one more like that so we're almost into the end of the journey

we've got to do some pretty challenging things don't you think I think we've built up into it all right excellent work so we're going to come to standing and let's go behind our chair now here's the thing right it's really hard with me behind my chair for you to see what I'm doing so I'm just going to step out from behind my chair so you can see me a little bit better but I want you to feel like you know standing behind the chair is great because you're going to have that full support of the chair

so we're going to place our weight into our left leg and I want you to cross that right ankle over that left ankle okay now lift nice and Tall through the spine Bend this knee and shoot your hips back okay so you're holding onto that chair it's giving you that support we have one more breath and then we're going to come up and unravel okay so now we're going to do that on the other side so put the weight into the other leg cross at the ankle Bend at supporting knee shoot your hips back behind you

and let your heart begin to fall forward go ahead and lift the heart and unravel so we're going to do that one more time and what I want you to try to think about is maybe walk your hands down the left the back of the chair so you're letting your heart fall a little further and if you don't have space for your face you know what I mean so you can come to the side of the chair or just take a couple of steps back so that you've got space okay put the weight into the left leg crop cross that right

ankle on in front pull the belly in Bend the supporting knee shoot the hips back now maybe you walk your hands down the side of that leg up the leg the side of the chair is what I'm trying to say so I just want you to make sure your hips are staying back you're just letting your heart fall a little further pushing the hips back is going to enhance the stretch one more breath go ahead and come up and let's unravel and do the other side okay bend that supporting knee shoot your hips back and just kind of make your way down so

I'm just kind of you know just kind of walking yourself down the back of that chair ooh feel the stretch man one more breath go ahead and roll it up okay so now that's a really really good version and I want you to stick with that version if you wish I am going to add one pretty significant add-on and again you just got to do it if it works for you so let's put the weight into that left leg now instead of Crossing ankle to ankle I'm going to bend my supporting knee a little bit and I want to bring this

ankle up so it's kind of ankle to leg all right so that standing knee is soft push your hips back and then let your heart begin to fall forward hold that chair this isn't balanced so don't worry about balance now it might be where you can even bring your hands to the floor one more breath grab the chair and roll up okay so go ahead and unravel and peek at me real quick here's the thing though so I've bent my knee and I've come down if you have your hands to the chair I mean to the floor excuse me what you

need to have is both hands on the floor equally so if you're feeling like you're having to compensate for that leg and like one hand is down and one hand is is up I would rather you go ahead and lift up a little bit hold on to the chair and have everything be symmetrical okay so let's go to the other side so remember you can cross ankle to ankle it's fine if you're with me we're going to be doing an ankle to knee cross here so we're going to bend that supporting knee and we're shooting our hips back

see I feel that already I mean I already feel it and you might find this side you can have a deeper stretch the other side not it's so common right to have one side be more or less willing than the other so if you want to begin to walk your hands down the leg the chair that's fine if you want to have your fingertips on the floor or your hands on the floor that's fine just make sure that you're symmetrical right so you're not compensating for one side or the other we have one more breath go ahead and grab that chair

begin to roll up this is not balance hold that chair this is not balance and unravel and come to standing how did that feel that's quite a stretch into those hips isn't it okay so now we're going to do a standing tree so we're going to place the weight into the leg next to the chair and we're going to create our little kickstand pull that belly in lift those pelvic floor muscles remember this is the key to balance we're going to release the chair and bring our hands to Heart now finding a spot in front of you to focus on that's not moving is a really good idea do you want to add your arms to the ceiling for those beautiful branches to our trees let's bring our hands back to Heart bring the hand down and Ries okay let's do the other side before we add on so weight is in to the leg next to the chair we're going to create our little kickstand here remember belly tied pelvic floor muscles lift it feels okay we're going to let go of that chair we're going to bring our hands to Heart I'm going to extend those arms up to the

ceiling finding that spot that's not moving focusing in on it one more breath bring your hands back to Heart release okay so we're going to stay on this side of the chair we're going to do it again and if you want the add-on instead of staying in kickstand you're going to bring your foot up it can come up to your calf or it can come up into the inner thigh it really doesn't matter to me or it can stay in kickstand fine remember belly tight okay are we ready here we go put the weight into the

leg next to the chair create your kickstand hold that chair belly tied pelvic floor muscles lift find that spot that's not moving bring your hands to Heart now if you're going to lift the leg let's do that now you choose and how to prepare exhale extend the arms up for the beautiful branches of those trees one more breath bring your hands back to Heart put the foot down mindfully remember we want to come out of it mindfully let's come to the other side put the weight into the leg next to the chair create your kickstand pull that

belly in bring your hands to Heart okay lift that foot up if you wish bring your arms up adding the branches to our beautiful trees we have one more breath here bring your hands back down to Heart and bring that foot down okay really really good so we're going to come behind our chair and we're going to do a heel toe and a heel toe all right so the legs are at an angle we've done this one before goddess pose pull the belly in bend your knees shoot your hips back so now we're going to release the chair

and we're going to take our one hand and place it on our belly and the other hand and place it on our heart see if you can get any deeper into that that goddess pose oh yeah we have one more breath here let's hold the chair straighten the legs take just a moment okay let's do it again bend the knees can you get any deeper see if you can get any deeper down into that goddess pose oh yeah let's let go of the chair and let's switch hands the other hand on the belly the other hand on the heart for three and two and one hold the chair straighten those legs and bring those feet in excellent work really really good okay so we're going to come to the right side of our chair and do a standing Sun salutation with a chair pose so bring your hands to Heart we've done this one before we're going to add the chair and we're going to add some twisting up we go to Mountain pose bring your hands to Heart come back up to Mountain pose and let's do our forward salute stretching through that spine nice and

long place your hands on your thighs let that heart fall forward for that supported forward fold tuck the chin and roll in it bring your hands to Heart let's reverse one dive up Mountain pose hands to Heart hands come back up inhale exhale dive it forward forward salute airplane arms stretch it out place your hands on your thighs let the heart fall forward okay now we're going to bend our knees we're going to bring our hands to heart shoot your hips back into chair pose feel that so I can wiggle my toes a little bit

one more breath and let's stand up and we're gonna do it one more time and add the twist up we go bring your hands to Heart come back up to Mountain pose dive forward forward salute airplane arms stretch it out come into your chair pose bend your knees shoot your hips back heart is lifted okay so this one is a pretty challenging pose all right so I want you to do what feels good to you we're going to twist towards our chair now I want you to look down at your feet lift your right heel off the mat

push that foot back revolved Crescent lunge so I'm twisting towards my chair my opposite leg is back behind me front knee is bent one more breath that back foot is going to come forward into a twist take the twist out stand up and release let's come to the other side I know it's challenging but hey we're almost done with our 28 days we can do this right bring your hands to Heart let's reverse Swan Dive up to Mountain pose bring your hands to heart look how far we've come up we go inhale to prepare exhale diving

forward forward salute air plate arms hands on thighs for that supported forward fold bring your hands to your heart bend your knees shoot your hips back into your chair pose belly is tight okay we got this let's twist our chair pose towards our chair look down at your feet lift your left heel up off the mat shoot that foot back behind you revolved Crescent lunge I know very challenging front knee is bent we're twisting towards our chair belly is tight one more breath here now listen bring the back foot forward first there's our chair pose twist twisted chair take the twist out stand up and release yay so so good all right let's come to seated we're going to sit back in our chair we're gonna move into shavasana pose place your hands lightly on your thighs close your eyes take a deep breath in and a full breath out a deep breath in and a full complete cleansing breath out start sooner take a moment to think back about all

you've done in your life you'll discover a lot more undertakings you now wish you had started sooner and hardly any you wish you had started later what can you learn from this your own experience demonstrates the value of starting sooner rather than later is there something you've been thinking about doing same learning mastering now is the time to stop thinking about it and start putting it into practice if it's worth doing it's worth starting sooner to get the most out of your effort and commitment start sooner

but perhaps you can't start until you've made sufficient preparations then start sooner on the preparations put as much time as possible on your side let go of your doubt and hesitation and start sooner take a deep breath in into full breath out drop your right ear towards your right shoulder reach up with the right hand give the head a gentle tug pressing that left hand down towards the floor release it drop your chin towards your chest reach up with the hands give the head a gentle tug release it

drop your left ear towards your left shoulder reach up with the left hand give the head a gentle tug pressing that right hand down towards the floor release it look out just slightly open your mouth if you want to stretch your jaw bring your hands to your heart

DAY 27

we're going to move forward in our chair making sure that spine is nice and long focusing just a few moments on that connection of the Mind the body and the breath thinking about having both feet on the floor and grounding each of those feet grounding our sits bones to the chair lifting up through our heart lowering those shoulders down out of the ears placing their hands lightly on the thighs let's lift those Palms up close your eyes connect to your breath just feel that natural inhalation and exhalation let's go ahead and elongate the breath so we're going to inhale a little more deeply and exhale a little more completely and just do that a few more times breathe normally bring your hands to your heart set your intentions for today's practice just one more breath here bring your hands back down to your thighs and open your eyes and we're going to roll at our shoulders ah up back and down right so just feel that maybe you move your head a little side to side and let's reverse it it's just a little opening for the shoulders and the neck and let's release that okay okay so let's do our Mountain pose we're

going to extend our arms down by our side Palms are facing out extending those fingers for a nice stretch go post arms squeeze those shoulder blades back behind you and extend let's bring our right hand to our chair and extend that left hand up oh that should feel really good and release let's do that whole thing again here we go Mountain pose nice long spine go post arms really feeling the openness in the chest here and extending our Mountain let's bring that left hand down try to touch the ceiling with that right

hand feeling that stretch and release very very good we'll do some pelvic tilts to do a little warm-up for the spine so I'm going to take my hip tips and rot them towards my shoulders all right and then I'm going to take those hip tips and I'm going to rock them towards the knees so the back is just a little you know Arch and then round so that's the hip tips to shoulders and hip tips to knees one more time feeling that movement in this lower spine right and up we go and release very good so move forward a

little forward in your chair and take those feet a little bit wider than hip distance now I'm going to hold on behind my on the seat of my chair behind my back and I'm going to let my knees fall to the right as you do that I want you to look over that left shoulder all right let's bring everything Center and then we're going to let our knees fall the other way and look the opposite direction and then we're going to come back Center okay so we got one little add-on here so we're going to drop our knees back to

the right I want you to pick your right foot and place it up on that left leg if that feels okay if you don't want to do that that's all right so get that feeling first then if it's if it's feeling okay you're going to turn and look over that left shoulder let's come Center remove that leg so windshield wiper knees we're going to let our knees fall to the left now we're going to pick that left foot up and place it up on top of that right leg I don't know about you but I feel that

quite a stretch now we're going to look over that right shoulder so just do whichever piece of this feels okay for you right don't ever feel like you've got to add anything on that doesn't feel good and face forward and release all right excellent work we're going to bring our forearms parallel to one another now this right arm we're going to do a half shoulder press up to the ceiling and then we're going to open our book so we're going to do a little movement for our shoulder joint and then we're going

to bring that arm forward bring your palm to face you and do a bicep curl and let's do the other side so it's a little half shoulder press up then we're going to open and then Palm faces you for a bicep curl so having the elbows bent let's do it again on the other side should be okay on your shoulder but just listen to your body right and if it want doesn't want you to open it all the way don't listen to what it's telling you then a little palm faces you for that bicep curl let's do the other side half shoulder

press I call this opening the book and a bicep curl and release okay so now we're going to do that instead of the half shoulder press we're going to do the full shoulder press so we're going to start one at one at a time and then we'll add both at the same time if it feels better for you to stick with the half shoulder press that's what you'll do all right arms parallel here we go full shoulder press bend the elbow open the book close the book bicep curl and let's do the other side full

shoulder press down we go open the book and bicep curl now we're going to do both arms at the same time are we ready here we go full shoulder press up bring it down open your book and close bicep curl and let's do that one more time full shoulder press up down we go open that book and bicep curl excellent work very very good so come forward in your chair now you're going to have your hands sitting here and then we're gonna lift this knee up and you're just going to bounce your hand onto that knee and then

we're going to switch sides bounce and up down and up hand is bouncing and up again bounce and up belly tight crown of the head lifts we're not leaning back now listen here we go two other side two switch sides two other side two switch sides two other side two last one like this we're going to add on from here and two now we're going four ready here we go four three two one switch sides four belly is tight crown of the head to the ceiling switch sides four three two one switch sides this is it last one

and release I don't know about you I know I felt that in my arms and I felt that in my legs abdominals were engaged all right very good so now we're going to do knee circles with a little ankle rotation so we're going to lift our right knee and I've got my hand right underneath so then I'm going to rotate that leg out then I'm going to bring it down and up and let's do that again out down around and up one more out down around and up now bring it in hold and this rotate the ankle reverse it

okay let's put that foot down we're going to the other side so we're going to bring it up first hold on the other hand can be holding the chair if that feels better for you belly tight crown of the head to the ceiling we're going to bring the knee out down around and up again out down around and up one more out down around and reverse it we got this keep going so we're just doing a little rotation for that hip joint right all right go ahead and stop grab the the behind the thigh extend the spine long

and let's rotate the ankle and reverse it and put that foot down okay so now what we're going to do is we're going to grab with our right arm we're going to hook right underneath that leg so I want a nice long spine crowd of the head to the ceiling this hand can hold if you want you can kind of hold on to that wrist or that hand now we're going to extend that leg and then we're going to release it we're going to extend and release extend and release now listen extend and hold pull your belly in let's reach up

and grab that leg give it just a little tug oh yeah bend the knee and put the foot down so the key to this one this leg hook series is not to lean back so we want to keep the crown of the head long make your abdominals work here okay so let's do the other side we're going to hook that leg over that arm you can hold on to that wrist nice long spine right here we go extend and bend extend and bend extend and bend one more extend and hold reach up and grab that leg give it just a little tug oh yeah don't lean back

belly tight bend the knee and put the foot on the floor okay great version stick with that version if you want to if you want to add on with me let's go to the other side we're going to hook it in nice long spine belly tight here we go extend and bend extend and bend extend and bend now extend hold reach up and grab now I want you to peek at where your toes are in relationship to the wall or the ceiling we're going to let go of the leg and I want you to see if you can keep your toes in that same position ready release oh yeah did it

fall down I know right hold one more breath bend the knife other side here we go look it around did I feel okay nice long spine belly tight this is a little abdominal work here Bend extend extend and bend I think I said it wrong extend and bend one more extend hold Reach Out grab give it just a little tug we're going to let go see if you can hold it up one more breath bend the knee and put this out so we have one final add-on to that okay let's hook it under all right so we're going to extend and we're going to hold reach up grab give

it a tug now we're going to let go and then we're going to bring the leg down and then we're going to lift it up bring the leg down and lift it up quadriceps belly bound and up one more down and up bend the knee put the foot on the floor are you leaning back I know it's hard not to think about lifting up through that spine last one last side let's do it extend okay reach up grab give it a little tug peek at where your toes are on that wall let go now we're going to go down and up down and up

down and up one more down and up bend the knee that one's hard leg hook series okay so the next series are good mornings and here we're going to be working into our abdominals and our side waist muscles so we're going to sit forward in our chair lean all the way back we don't ever get to do this right we're leaning back and we're resting Cross Your Arms over your chest take a deep breath in and as you inhale as you exhale lift yourself up and come into seated so your knees are bent your feet are going to stay on the

floor just make your abdominals use the do the work inhale exhale up we go now your back is going to touch the chair as you come back but you're not resting and up we go and back so the back to the chair but don't rest and up we go and back okay go ahead and lean back take a moment now the hands are going to come behind the head so here's our first little add-on inhale to prepare exhale up we go and back we go inhale to prepare and up and back ready up now as you come back and make those abs do the work don't pull on that neck up

we go and back one more up we go and back so here's the final little add-on before we do the sideways is we extend our legs long feet have to stay down okay so they're going to want to lift up don't let that happen that just means your hips are trying to help okay let's start across on our chest inhale exhale up we go you feel the difference right inhale back we go exhale lift it up inhale back we go exhale lift it up back we go now we're going to go straight to the hands behind the head ready here we go

back and up oh yeah are those feet coming up don't matter back make your abs do the work if the feet are coming up it means your hip flexors are helping we don't want that we want the abdominals to do the work ah and up let's do one more back and okay really really good so now we're going to do just a little bit for that side waist okay so we're going to bend those knees Let's cross here first we're going to twist and Center so I'm extending one leg and I'm twisting the other way and Center

and twist and Center and twist and Center again twist and Center last one twist now bring your hands behind your head twist and Center and twist and Center twist come Center and Center last time we're going to do both sides though and Center last time twist and Center excellent excellent work okay so we're going to come to standing and we're going to come to the right side of our chair and get ready for Eagle pose so go ahead and come to standing I'm going to give you various options okay so if you're like yeah I don't know

about Eagle pose just just know that I'm going to give you some options so the first thing we're going to do is we're going to keep our feet on the floor you're like hi yay right so we're not going to do balance to begin with we're just going to do a little bit of of work into the side waist so right through the center of the body okay so we're going to come up and we're going to do wrist to wrist and then we're going to twist to the right and then we're going to come Center

and we're going to twist to the left and we're going to come Center we're going to lift up and center and we're going to go down and center now put the other wrist on top twist to the left come Center twist to the right and come Center lift up and Center and down and Center okay really good now bring your arms out to the side that's doing Palms to face up you're going to take your right arm on top okay and then you're going to bend your elbows backs of the Palms together or the fronts of the Palms are together

lifting up okay are we ready let's go to the right and Center let's go to the left and Center we're going to go up and center and we're going to go down and Center let's unravel and then go the other side backs of the hands are together or the fronts lift up forearms away from the face turn to the right left excuse me and Center turn to the right and Center Arms up and Center Arms down and Center and release okay so now we're going to add just lifting one foot up okay so we're going to come into that eagle knee now

let's just cross wrist to wrist if that feels okay so we're going to bring that knee up so I've got my weight into the leg next to the chair and I'm going to bring this knee up my belly is super tight here okay Let's cross the wrist to wrist oh yeah just one more breath here unravel put that foot down and we're going to go to the other side okay so lift the other knee up cross wrist to wrist one more breath and release okay so the very final piece of this is we're going to do the actual

Eagle ledge so what that is hold your chair we're going to bring that knee up and we're going to let it slide down our standing leg now maybe you go all the way down where those toes touch creating a little kickstand or maybe you don't right either is fine oh okay excuse me so let's put our weight into the leg next to the chair let's bring that knee up Flex the foot let that leg slide down the standing leg okay create your kickstand if you want let go of the chair so we're going to cross wrists to wrist

to start with beautiful equal pose right here one more breath okay let's unravel take a moment now if you want the final add-on we're getting remember how we did those Eagle arms where we did here so we're going to do that all right let's do it put the weight into the leg next to the chair bring that knee up slide it down belly tight okay so bring those arms out wide now you're going to cross right arm on Top Bend at the elbows back so the hands are together or the fronts of the Palms are

together lift your arms up forearms away from the face Eagle arms Eagle pose three two one unravel and unravel excellent work okay we gotta do the other side though so we've done most of it on the other side we just go to that last little piece okay so I want you to be on this side of the chair we're going to put the weight into the leg next to the chair go ahead and bring that knee up okay let's hold the chair first slide that leg down get the feeling of that eagle lit legs right so if you want to create the

kickstand with your toes on the floor that's fine if you don't that's okay too all right are we got that feeling we've got the leg set okay we're gonna let go of the chair let's go and uh let's cross wrist to wrist to start with just to kind of get the feeling of it here before we add the eagle arms belly is super tight one more breath here let's unravel and take a moment okay let's do the whole thing we got this put the weight into the leg next to the chair bring that opposite knee up

Let the heel slide down that standing leg create the kickstand if you want your toes can be down or not pull that belly in find that spot that's not moving bring those arms out wide we're going to cross left arm on top Bend at the elbows back to the Palms together or fronts of the Palms are together lift your arms up forearms away from the face one more breath unravel and uh oh my goodness standing Eagle pose super challenging you guys did Fabulous we're gonna turn now and we're going to face the seat of our chair and your hip

feet are going to be hip distance apart we're going to move into camel pose with a cat and a cow so I'm going to take my hands I've got one hand on each side of my spine right in the small of my back my shoulders are down out of my ears my heart is lifted I'm just going to push my hips forward so this creates a little bit of a backbend do you see that just a little bit of a back bend not much one more breath now pull your belly button in towards your spine release hinge forward place your hands in the

seat of the chair bring your weight forward so my shoulders are right over my wrists drop the belly lift the heart lift the hips into cow pose pull the belly button in towards the spine tuck the chin around the shoulders and come into cat pose do that again dropping the belly lifting the heart lifting the hips rounding the spine rounding the shoulders tucking the chin and moving into cat Cow pose excuse me cat folks all right let's go ahead and bend the knees and come up into standing position okay we're gonna do that one more time

all right so let's place the hands right here one on each side of the spine shoulders are down squeezing those shoulder blades back behind you all right shoulders are down into the ears squeezing the shoulder blades behind now we're just going to push those hips forward now if it feels okay and you're like yeah that one was pretty good maybe you push your hips a little further forward and if you look up there is a candle pose another version right just a little deeper stretch into camel only do this

if it feels okay on your back right one more breath let's come up slowly belly tight come back into that and this to that cat Cow again hands are in the seat of the chair bring the weight forward drop the belly lift the heart lift the hips cow pose pull the belly button to spine round the shoulders tuck the chin into your cat pose let's do that again dropping the belly lifting the heart lifting the hips and then pull the belly button in rounding the shoulders into your cat pose come back to neutral spine bend the

knees and roll up excellent work so we're going to take our neat leg next to the chair and we're going to place that foot right under the chair bend that knee so that the leg touches the chair opposite leg steps back heel is down bring your hips forward to face the chair and bend that front knee pull the belly in lengthen through the tailbone bring the hands to Heart inhale exhale extend that arm up for a beautiful Warrior One pose ha we have one more breath here now starting with this outside hand you're

going to Windmill around to that Warrior Two all right very good let's flip that Palm up and back and we're going to come back to our Warrior Two now you're going to straighten this front leg okay I want the upper body we're moving into triangle upper body comes over the chair it comes over the chair and oh see how this hip is hiking up now bring that hand into the chair and lift up oh my goodness that this that feels so good nice stretch for that front leg you feel it High make sure your chest is open hands

are up in the air you've got wrist shoulder shoulder wrist and Alignment right one more breath let's bend that front knee and press back up into that Warrior Two let's flip that Palm up and back now come back to your Warrior Two straighten the front leg upper body moves over that chair moves over the chair moves over the chair hand down lifting up into that triangle pose one more breath bend that front knee press up into Warrior Two reverse your Warrior up and back last time through back to Warrior Two

straighten the front leg move the upper body over that chair place the hand down into that triangle pose that front leg is straight it wants to bend don't let it there's that inner thigh stretching right oh yeah you got this one more breath bend that front knee press back up into Warrior Two and release oh yeah you feel that okay we gotta do the other side all right so we're going ahead and place that foot under the chair remember you want to bend the knee feel the chair all right other other leg steps back heel is

down hips turn towards your chair bend that front knee pull that belly in tight lengthen through that tailbone bring your hands to Heart in how to prepare exhale extend the arms to the ceiling for the beautiful Warrior One pose oh yeah hanging out here for a couple more breaths now we're going to Windmill to that Warrior Two flip this front Palm up and back back to Warrior Two straighten your front leg upper leg upper body is lengthening over the chair all over the chair it just won't go any further then you let your hand slide

down to the chair and open up into your triangle pugs you can look up if you want to you don't have to you can look out bend that front knee press up into Warrior Two flip that front Palm up and back reverse your Warrior back to Warrior Two ready straight in the front leg over the chair we go over the chair we go and one more and then down into triangle ha make sure your wrist shoulder shoulder wrist or in alignment so don't don't be here okay lifting up bend that front knee press back to Warrior Two

flip the Palm up and back we've got this ready back to Warrior Two I know final was straight in the front leg upper body over the chair over the chair it won't go any further then you put that hand down lifting up I feel my inner thigh I don't know about you one more breath bend that front knee press back into that Warrior Two one more breath let's come to seed it that was really really good good work okay so I'm going to take my right knee and open it I'm going to let my left knee fall down towards the the floor for

a crescent lunge lifting that heart up it should feel good after all that worked just a nice little stretch release it and let's do that again so back of the kneecap up towards the ceiling lifting up through the heart one more breath here and release let's face forward same leg extends out lengthen through the spine let the heart fall forward keep that back flat tuck the chin roll it up one more time nice long spine heart Falls forward and roll it up okay let's do the other side leg opens up this leg falls down towards

the floor push that foot back lift your heart ah release it and then back of the kneecap up towards the ceiling heart stays lifted one more breath here and release face forward let's extend this leg out in front of us toes to the ceiling lengthen and hinge pyramid pose tuck the chin and roll it up and we're gonna do that one more time nice long spine heart Falls forward ah very good okay let's move into shavasana pose we're gonna lean back in our chair hands are going to rest lightly on the thighs

flip the Palms up towards the ceiling take a deep breath in and as you exhale close or soften those eyes achieve what you desire the results you get are not simply a function of what you desire they're a function of what your desires inspire you to do on its own without any further action setting a goal is meaningless for a goal to matter it must prompt you to make some change in the way you live your life what you desire in your personal life your career in your level of physical fitness what commitment are you willing to make

what actions are you willing to take to fulfill those desires it can be fun to dream and wish what's a whole lot more satisfying and a whole lot more work is to achieve what you desire fortunately you have the power to transform dreams into reality you can think you can act you can learn adapt and persist you're never too old too young too rich or too poor to set a meaningful goal and work toward it no matter your situation it's always a great thing to do take a deep breath in and a full breath out

drop your right ear towards your right shoulder reach up with the right hand give the head a gentle tug pressing that left hand down towards the floor release it drop your chin towards your chest reach up with the hands give the head a gentle tug release it drop your left ear towards your left shoulder reach up with the left hand give the head a gentle tug pressing that right hand down towards the floor release it look up just slightly open your mouth if you want to stretch your jaw bring your hands to your heart

DAY 28

I'm so glad you joined me today so today is day 28 of our 28 day chair yoga journey together I am so thankful that you've chosen to go on this journey with me it's been a very powerful experience for me personally and I hope for you too and I also hope that you feel a sense of accomplishment for sticking to it and seeing your commitment to the end so we are going to start seated we'll move into a standing warrior pose we are going to be using the block today so you know if you have that block that's great if you substitute a large book for it that's great if you don't have it don't worry about it it's fine so let's go ahead if you have it set it down there under your chair remember if you'd click subscribe I appreciate it it's free leave me a comment and let's get started so we're going to sit up nice and tall in our chair right we're moving forward in our seat we're not leaning back

take a moment to focus on that mind and body and breath grounding our feet to the Earth grounding our sits bones to the chair lifting her heart lowering our shoulders hands on the thighs flip the Palms up close the breath I close the breath close the eyes and connect to your breath just feeling your inhalation and exhalation noticing that breath we're going to move that breath down into the diaphragm as we inhale the belly extends we're filling those lungs from the bottom up and as we exhale we actively pull the

belly button in towards the spine pushing the air up and out of the lungs do that a couple of more times and breathe normally now we're going to continue with our diaphragmatic breath we're going to inhale to four counts and then exhale to five counts it'll be something like this inhale two three four exhale two three four five inhale two three four exhale two three four five and breathe number nine bring your hands to your heart set your intentions for today's practice one more breath here bring your hands back down to your

thighs and open your eyes we're going to let our right ear fall towards our right shoulder reach back and grab the chair squeeze your shoulder blades back behind you and let that ear fall a little further if it works okay for you let's drop our chin towards our chest see if you can maintain the squeeze of the shoulder blades back behind you and then we're going to draw that left ear to that left shoulder squeezing the chair now release the hands behind you leave the head in that extension feeling the neck stretching and then bring the head up okay excellent work so now we're going to move into Cobra pose to child's pose so what I'd like for you to do is grab your block and just place it between your feet okay for now you'll see why here in a second now we're going to move back in our chair and what I want you to do is to place we're going to move into Cobra pose first so you're going to place the inside of the arms right on the outside of the leg of the leg the outside of the back of the chair

all right do you see kind of what I'm doing there so I've got the inside of my arms to the outside of the back of the chair now I'm not really leaning back so I'm not here resting I want you to think about lifting up through the heart opening up through the chest so the hands are just kind of resting here on the side look up slightly so Cobra pose seated Cobra pose we have one more breath here now we're going to move into child's pose so I'm going to let my belly come forward and I'm just going to drop my hands between

my legs and kind of let my head fall down all right tuck the chin and roll it up okay so that's generally what we're doing now what we're going to be doing is the with the block is we're going to try to get our head a little bit lower and place our hands on the Block okay if it feels okay if that doesn't feel good for you then you're just going to stay right here and there's nothing wrong with this child's pose it's absolutely fine let's do that again so we're gonna

we're coming back just a little bit but not leaning back on the back of the chair place the inside of the arms on the outside of the chair back squeeze your shoulder blades behind you lift your heart looking up there's that Cobra pose so it's a nice hard lifting opening right so we're hoping opening up through that chest one more breath now pull your belly in hinge forward place your hands between your legs now see if you can let your heart fall any further and maybe your hands go on to the block

let that head fall if that feels okay roll up into seated position okay we're gonna do that one more time here we go cobra looking up oh yeah feel that stretch through the sternum one more breath and down we go into that child's pose hands to the block if that feels okay for you letting yourself just kind of hang out here between your legs hands are resting on that block for support if we don't have the block the hands can be resting on your legs or on the floor one more breath and roll it up into seated position okay excellent work let's grab our block now again if you don't have the block don't worry about it it's fine but the lock is in my right hand and my other hand is up at goal post arms so I'm going to bring this hand across I'm going to grab my block and then I'm going to grab it and open now my other arm is going to come across grab the block and open don't bring the block to the hand make the hand go all the way to the block add the block and open just a little seated twist here right

grab that block and open one more time on each side bring the arm across grab the block and open and we're going to do the other side grab the block and open and release okay very good so the next series is going to be a sun salutation which I know we've done a lot this time we're going to move with our forward fold we're going to use our block to give us some support so I'm going to place that block in that tall number three position right between our feet if you don't have the block you're

going to be using your legs for support as you walk down okay so that's fine Bring Your Hands to heart so we're going to reverse one dive all the way up to Mountain pose and we're going to bring our hands to Heart then we're going to come back up to Mountain pose and we're going to come forward salute airplane arms stretching through the spine all right let's start with our supported forward follow place your forearms on the thighs and let the heart fall forward tuck the chin and roll it up so you

should feel your back working and stretching there hands to Heart let's do that again just like that up we go to Mountain pose bring your hands to Heart we're going to come back to Mountain dive forward forward salute airplane arms stretching through the spine supported forward fold let the heart fall forward tuck the chin and roll it up adding on hands to Heart here we go big circle up bring your hands to Heart inhale as you come up if you want to add the breath exhale forward salute our plane arms we got this let's do that for

uh supported forward fold okay now instead of having your hands on your thighs you're going to reach down put your hands on the Block and let that heart fall a little further there's the back tuck the chin and roll it up bring your hands to your heart okay now we're going to move that block to the number two position and if you're using your legs you're just going to take your hands down a little further on the legs ready big circle up we go Mountain pose bring your hands to Heart add that breath if you want to back up your Mountain pose forward salute airplane arms stretching all right forward fold now take your hands off the legs place them on the Block let the heart fall a little further tuck the chin roll it up bring your hands to your heart let's move that block to the number one position are we ready big circle up we go Mountain pose bring your hands to heart back to Mountain pose forward salute airplane arms forward fold all right are we ready move the hands to the block let that heart fall a little further

touch the chin roll it up to seated now if you want to just do it without the block just let that block back a little bit under your chair bring your hands to Heart big circle up we go Mountain pose bring your hands to heart back up we go forward salute our plane arms stretching all right forward fold let's start here let that heart Begin to Fall now if you want you're going to bring your hands to the floor now if it feels okay you're going to tuck your chin and you're going to look under your chair

we have one more breath here now come up slowly go ahead and place your hands back on the thighs for support roll yourself up nice and slow take your time here I don't want you to get this ah how did that feel excellent work we're going to move into gate pose next so let's all move to the right side of our chair so you've got I got one cheek on and One Cheek off and let's extend that right leg out to the side so inner and outer thighs we're going to be stretching and working here so you're up

on the edge of that foot okay let's extend that left arm to the ceiling right at the arm is on that leg and it's going to slide down as we close our gate now we're going to come up we're going to place this hand on the chair lengthen that right arm and open that gate bringing that hand down to the chair extend close that gate make sure you're nice and long through the spine before you bend up we go place the hand on the chair opposite hand extends and open and we're going to do one more let's do

it extend lean up we go opposite arm extends and leans and up we go and release oh yeah that feel pretty good ready for the other side let's do it we're gonna scoot over the other side of that chair lengthen that other leg out all right let's extend that right arm up and close our gate up we go hand to the chair extend and lean up we go opposite side extend and let that hand slide down the leg as you close that gate up we go lengthen and hinge we've only had one more on each side we got this up we go little flow here right we're moving through down the hand goes to the chair opposite arm extends and and up we go all right really really good work is that feeling pretty good A little stretch feel like we warmed up okay we're going to take our right knee and we're going to open it up and we're going to move into our Crescent lunge okay so this knee falls down towards the floor bring your hands to your heart okay so we're going to bring those hands up to the ceiling now you're going to Windmill and face me

take your hands back up to the ceiling and you're going to Windmill and face the other way hands back to the ceiling let's squeeze our shoulder blades behind us in goal post arms looking up slightly bring the hands down to the chair release and take just a little break okay let's do the other side okay so we're going to take this left knee and we're going to open it up right knee is going to fall down towards the floor okay lifting your heart out Bring Your Hands to Heart now we're going to extend the arms up to

the ceiling and we're going to rotate face me hands back to the ceiling rotate and face over the back of your chair hands to the ceiling we're going to squeeze our shoulder blades behind us go post arms looking up slightly hands back to the ceiling bring your hands back down to the chair face forward and release okay so we're going to add one thing to that series and that is we're going to slip our hips off of the chair and move through that sequence okay so you don't have to you can keep your hips right on

that chair and that's fine so let's take that knee and open it wide let that knee fall down towards the floor so here we are in our Crescent lunge right now I'm just going to slip my hips off of the chair bring your hands to heart so make sure your abdominals are tight your spine is long lengthen the hands to the ceiling now you're going to Windmill and face me hands to the ceiling Windmill and face over your chair hands to the ceiling goal post arms squeeze your shoulder blades behind you look up

hands to the ceiling bring your hands back to the chair slip your hips back on and face forward okay let's do the other side here we go bring that knee out opposite knee falls down towards the floor push that foot back behind you okay are we ready slip those hips off that chair I know right I gotcha bring your hands to Heart all right hands to the ceiling we go Windmill and face me belly tight up we go windmilling face over the seat of your chair up we go go post arms squeeze your shoulder blades behind look up slightly hands to the ceiling bring your hands to the chair slip your hips back on and a spoiler okay doing okay it's come to stand so I want to finish along with a tree pose right so we're gonna do that full tree and we're going to start in kickstands so we're going to put the weight next to the that's next to the in put the weight into the leg that's next to the chair I'll get that out here in a second create your kickstand so my heel is up against the standing ankle right belly is tight bring your hands to heart now remember

belly tight pelvic floor muscles lift find a spot that's not moving focus in on it add to branches to your trees bring your hands back down to Heart and grab the chair and release okay so we're going to stay on this side of the chair and we're going to go ahead and add that lifting leg so all you'll do is you can place your foot against your quad or Shin or you can lift it up and bring it in to the inside of that leg I don't care it'd been matter to me either one is fine okay or you can stay in

kickstand it's fine too all right so let's all start in kickstand so my ankles right up against that uh my heel is up against that standing ankle remember belly tight we're going to let go of the chair bring your hands to Heart now if you want you're going to lift that foot up let's add our branches to our trees belly tight we have one more breath here bring your hands back to a heart put your foot down mindfully we're going to the other side just we can stay on this side of the chair so create your kickstand first

bring your hands to your heart let's leave our foot down and kickstand to start with extend those arms up towards the ceiling adding the branches to our beautiful trees bring their hands back to Heart put the foot down for just a moment okay are we ready back to kickstand now if you wish lift your foot up add the branches to the trees one more breath here bring your hands back down to your heart and put that foot down mindfully excellent very good okay so we're gonna move into a quadruped series so I'm going to take a little step back

from my chair okay so I'm not too close to it so whenever I hinge I want to be able to bring my hands to the chair and bring my weight forward okay so if I'm too too close to it I don't really have this you know where I can bring my weight forward you want the shoulders right over wrists okay so I encourage you to just look down I may look out at the camera just so I can peek at you but don't don't feel like you you need to turn your head you can look straight down at the chair okay so we're gonna start by taking our outside arm right so your right arm extend it out now the opposite leg is going to come back behind you and you're up on those toes okay so here is version one of our quadruped your abdominals are engaged pretty tightly let's bring that hand down and bring the foot forward and then we're going to go to the other side okay so we're extending the arm is extended out the foot is back behind the toes are on the floor and back we go okay let's bend the knees and roll up and check in so how are we

feeling on that one okay so we're going to add on a couple of things here so hinge forward hands into the chair bringing the weight forward wrists to ride over I'm sorry shoulders are right over wrists okay okay so let's start let's extend that arm out the opposite leg back now instead of keeping the toes on the floor we're going to lift that leg up Flex the foot and I want you to push that foot back behind you put the arm push the arm out in front of you belly stays tight here one more breath come back Center we're

going straight to the other side here we go extend start with toes down then lift that leg up Flex the foot that's in the air push your foot towards the wall behind you push the fingertips towards the wall in front of you one more breath bring your hand down bring your foot down bend the knees and roll up okay everything feeling all right you're feeling like okay last little piece we're going to add one more thing on all right are we ready let's hinge forward place the hands in the seat of the chair

bring the weight forward all right let's extend the arm and the opposite leg is back now we're going to lift that leg up and I want you to cross it back behind you bring your hand back down to the chair turn and look at your back toes so we're adding in a little twist to our quadruped just one more breath here take the twist out bring that leg and put that foot on the floor can we go straight to the other side let's do it extend the arm first then put the leg back behind you toes down first now Flex the foot lift

that leg up pushing the foot into the wall behind you the fingertips to the wall in front of you now I'm going to take the leg and I'm going to bring it back behind and I'm going to put my hand back in the chair and I'm going to turn and I'm going to look at that back those back toes just one more breath go ahead and face forward bring that foot around bend the knees roll up into a standing position okay excellent so now grab your block if you have it and place it right here by your chair now if you don't have your block you're just going to use the seat of the chair and then if you want a little more you can walk your hands down your legs okay so let's come back just a smidge feet or hip distance apart okay now I'm going to hinge forward so we're moving into a forward fold I don't know if I even said that this is a forward fold Series so your hands can be on the in the seat of the chair maybe you let your heart fall a little further for a little more hamstring stretch or maybe you put your hands on the Block

and let that heart fall forward or maybe your hands are on your legs so you've got some options here see if you can let your head fall this is full version of a standing forward fold we have one more breath let's Bend our knees and we're going to roll up into standing hold that chair checking in how's that feel okay so now we're going to just move that block down into that flattest position and we're going to do that again okay now what will happen is we're going to get down and we're going to have our

hands on the on the Block and then we're going to see how it feels can we move the block away and put our hands on the floor okay just we're going to see how that feels if you want to keep the hands on the block that's okay all right are we ready let's hinge forward we got this place the hands on the Block remember they can be in the chair or they can be holding on to the legs if you don't have that block it's absolutely fine and if you want to keep the block High that's okay too right use you know use

your own discretion here what feels good for you okay so now I'm just going to hang out here for a couple more breaths see how that's feeling then maybe slide that block away and place your hands on the mat or on the floor right let that head fall keep the legs straight so we don't want to start bending the knees to get the hands down right I would much rather you have your hands up higher but the legs straight so that we're stretching the hamstring here all right let's bend the knees and roll

up hold on to that chair checking in how did that feel okay everybody all right so the very last thing we're going to add to this series is Ragdoll so when you're down what's going to happen is you're going to grab your elbows we're going to bend our knees and then you'll feel it more in the back so right now we're getting a lot of hamstring stretch right you're going to feel it more in the back okay rag doll all right so let's go ahead pick your version of forward fall doesn't matter whichever version and I'm going to grab my block I'm going to use my block this time letting that head fall okay so now to start Ragdoll I want you to bend your knees pretty generously let that heart fall a little further grab the elbows and then we're going to hang out here in ragdoll now nod your head yes if you wish you don't have to feels good to me shake your head no nod your head yes all right drop the hands back down to the block bend the knees or keep the knees bent really roll up hold your chair if you

may be a little a little light-headed from being in that uh inversion right and release all right how did that feel pretty good okay so we're just gonna you can place your block in the seat of your chair if you want to all that does is it lifts the seat of the chair up a little bit higher or you can just set it aside right so whatever you want to do I'm going to use my block so now I'm going to take my feet I've moved a little bit further forward and I'm going to take my feet a good the width of the chair legs maybe a little

bit more and I want your toes to point forward okay so this isn't goddess where our toes are pointing at a at a diagonal the toes are going to point forward pull that belly in okay now we're going to do a forward follow just like we've been doing and let's place our hands on the block or in the seat of the chair doesn't matter so we're going to bend our right knee and we're going to feel the inner thigh stretching on that left leg now we're going to come up and we're going to bend the other knee and feel

the inner thighs stretching and come up and bend come up and bend that other knee and go ahead and roll up and take just a little break okay so straddle forward fold now the one thing we're going to add to that is just a rotation okay so here I am and I'm going to bend one knee so I'm bending this knee and then I'm going to rotate the opposite direction okay and then I'm going to come Center and then we'll Bend and I'm going to rotate all right does that make sense okay so let's

go ahead and do our heel toe out so our legs our feet are the width of the chair legs or maybe a little more if that feels okay all 10 toes are pointing This Way Forward pull your belly in hinge forward place the hands on that on that block or chair doesn't matter okay so we're going to bend one knee and then we're going to revolve the opposite direction okay so you're opening up so if you've got your left knee bent your opening to the right okay and then we're going to come Center then we're going to bend the other knee and we're going to open the opposite direction so stacking those ribs one set of ribs are stacking on top of the other straighten the leg put the hand back on the chair open up bending that opposite knee placing the hand on the chair bend the other knee and open place the hand on the chair straighten both legs he'll toe your feet in together and release excellent work very good so we're going to add on a little bit from our yesterday's work with triangle and we're going to add our block so a

block is going to help us out again you can just use your chair just like we did yesterday but if you want a little bit more we're going to we're going to be using our our block okay so the first thing we're going to do is set our block on it on the end and we're going to put it on the inside of that foot okay so take that foot under the chair remember bending the knee take that opposite leg and step it back hips face forward bend that front knee so you see kind of where my block is bring your hands to Heart

okay belly tied extending through the spine tailbone is long inhale to prepare exhale up to that Warrior one now we're going to rotate around to that Warrior Two we've done this when we know it right let's go ahead and reverse our Warrior now we're going to come back to Warrior Two we're going to straighten our front leg upper body is going to come up over that chair over the chair over the chair now instead of coming into the seat of the chair like we did yesterday is going to come to the block now you can't let

yourself sink down into this right so I want you to lifting up through the chest relaxing to this bad glute so relax that let those hips come around one more breath bend that front knee come back to that Warrior Two okay so now straighten that front leg so we're gonna now we're going to take the block and we're going to move it to the outside of the Hat foot okay let's bring your hips back around get ready for that Warrior one bending that front knee so my blocks now on the outside of that leg bring your

hands to Heart bring your belly in lengthen through your tailbone okay ready inhale tip repair exhale extend the arms up to that Warrior one let's move to our Warrior Two reverse our Warrior up and back back to Warrior Two straighten your front leg upper body over the left over the chair over the chair over the chair now hand comes to the seat of the chair or it comes to that back see how much more you're open you have to open to grab that block it's just a little different right providing a little more opportunity to open through that chest this hand is up towards the ceiling for three two one bend the front knee press up Warrior Two and release excellent okay grab your butt let's come to the other side so first of all I'm going to place the block on the inside of that leg that foot right so bend that knee make sure that that uh that you can touch the chair step back hips are forward bend the front knee bring the hands to Heart okay belly is tight right lengthen through the tailbone inhale here exhale extend those arms up

to the ceiling ready we're going to Windmill to that Warrior Two flip the Palm up and back and then we're going to come back to our Warrior Two straighten the front leg upper body over the chair over the chair further then we're going to bring the hand to the seat of the chair or to the block oh yeah you feel that I feel it front leg right a lot of stretch one more breath bend that front knee press back up into that Warrior Two flip the Palm up and back to Warrior Two reach down and grab that block place it

on the outside of that leg bring those hips around Warrior one bring around to that Warrior Two flip the Palm up and back to reverse our Warrior we've got this back to Warrior Two straighten the front leg upper body comes over the chair over the chair now place the hand down in the seat of the chair or back to that back block I know it's quite the opening isn't it feeling that front leg stretching one more breath bend the front knee press back to that Warrior Two very least you guys did fabulous let's go ahead and have a seat

hi all right let's move into shavasana pose we're gonna lean back in our chair hands are going to rest lightly on the thighs flip the Palms up to the ceiling take a deep breath in and a full breath out close the eyes elevated perspective keep the little things little pay attention to the details but don't let those small matters grab your emotions and run away with them it's easy to expand a small disappointment into a dark cloud that lingers over your awareness fortunately it's just as easy to elevate

your perspective When A disruption or disappointment pops up quickly create some distance from it Envision yourself suddenly flying up to a thousand feet or fifteen thousand and consider the view from there from an elevated perspective you can see much more than whatever is frustrating you you can see the full extent of your resources positive possibilities hopes dreams and best expectations rather than obsessing over a monetary thorn in your side remind yourself of your most treasured values find fresh energy and enthusiasm to help you keep the small disappointments in their place refuse to be deterred from all the good you can do from an elevated perspective Focus your efforts on supporting and advancing what truly means the most take a deep breath in and a full breath out drop the right ear towards the right shoulder we check with the right hand give the head a gentle tug pressing that left hand down towards the floor release it drop your chin towards your chest reach up with the hands give the head a gentle tug release it

drop your left ear towards your left shoulder reach up with the left hand give the head a gentle tug pressing that right hand down towards the floor release it look out just slightly open your mouth if you want to stretch your jaw bring your hands to your heart.

so I hope you feel a sense of accomplishment because I know how hard you have worked and you know it takes discipline and willingness to stick to it to make it to the end of this chair yoga Journey

Conclusion

In the conclusion of our 28-Day Chair Yoga for Seniors book, we have embarked on a transformative journey together, exploring the many benefits of chair yoga for seniors. From increased flexibility and strength to improved mental well-being and overall health, this gentle practice has proven to be a powerful tool in enhancing the lives of seniors everywhere.

Throughout this 28-day challenge, we have learned a variety of chair yoga poses and techniques designed to cater to the unique needs and abilities of seniors. We have also discovered the importance of mindfulness and breath awareness, which have helped to create a strong foundation for our practice.

As we conclude this book, we encourage you to continue your chair yoga practice and to share your newfound knowledge with others. Remember to always listen to your body and modify the poses as needed to ensure a safe and enjoyable experience.

In the words of a wise yogi, "Yoga is not about touching your toes, it's about what you learn on the way down." So, as you continue your journey with chair yoga, embrace the lessons learned and the growth experienced along the way.

We hope this book has provided you with the tools and inspiration to lead a more active, balanced, and fulfilling life. May your practice continue to bring you joy, peace, and strength, and may you always find comfort and serenity in the embrace of your chair. Namaste.

Please wait, Your Review is Very Important…

Dear Reader,

I hope this message finds you well. Thank you for choosing to read the 28 Day Chair Yoga for Seniors to Lose Weight. Your feedback is incredibly valuable to me, and I would love to hear your thoughts on the book. Whether you've just started, are halfway through, or have finished reading, your perspective matters.

Your feedback is immensely appreciated and will help me enhance future works.

Thank you for taking the time to share your thoughts on 28 Day Chair Yoga for Seniors to Lose Weight. Your support means the world to me.

Happy reading!

Carol Bolden

Bonus: Free Video Tutorials

Full video course on the 28 day challenge (playlist)

Kindly type in the link below:

http://tinyurl.com/2zwajeu9

OR

Scan the QR code below

www.ingramcontent.com/pod-product-compliance
Lightning Source LLC
Chambersburg PA
CBHW080718260726
48660CB00010B/3583